Carol Harris has specialized in helping people to achieve their goals. She is founder of pc, and specializes in the development of people and organizations. Carol is qualified in Impression Management and is Chair of the Association for Neuro-Linguistic Programming. She works with both individual and corporate clients and has helped many people to get results through following her approach to weight control. Carol is also the author of *The Elements of NLP*.

Think Yourself Slim

A Unique Approach to Weight Loss

CAROL HARRIS

ELEMENT
Shaftesbury · Dorset
Boston · Massachusetts
Melbourne · Victoria

© Element Books Limited 1999
Text © Carol Harris 1999

First published in the UK in 1999 by
Element Books Limited
Shaftesbury, Dorset SP7 8BP

Published in the USA in 1999 by
Element Books, Inc.
160 North Washington Street, Boston, MA 02114

Published in Australia in 1999 by
Element Books Limited
and distributed by Penguin Australia Limited
487 Maroondah Highway, Ringwood,Victoria 3134

Cover design by Slatter-Anderson
Illustrated by David Woodroffe
Typeset by Footnote Graphics
Printed and bound in Great Britain by Caledonian
International Book Manufacturing Ltd, Glasgow

British Library Cataloguing in Publication data available

ACKNOWLEDGEMENTS

I would to thank:

Paul Harris for helping with the research on this book;
Dawn Marie Wedlock, Principal of the Fitness
Education Foundation of the Aerobics and Fitness
Association of Great Britain, for providing some of the
technical information on exercise;
The Institute for Optimum Nutrition for assisting with
dietary information;
Professor Gomer Williams for contributing to my own
personal fitness.

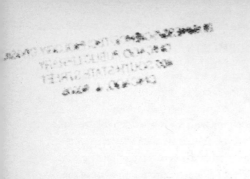

CONTENTS

PREFACE

Several years ago, I was looking at some wallpaper. It had a floral design and I noticed that some of the flowers on it were roses. As I had worked a good deal with thinking techniques, it occurred to me it would be interesting to see if I could imagine the smell of those roses, even though they were only pictures. I found it was quite easy to smell them.

My mind then turned to the issue of weight and what makes people overeat, or eat the 'wrong' things. It occurred to me that some people eat because the smell and taste they imagine for the food tempts them. I thought back to the roses. I realized that when someone imagined the smell and taste of a particular food and was then drawn to eat it, they could substitute another smell and taste in their imagination, for example lemons instead of chocolate. Instead of eating the original food, they could then either eat something healthier or avoid eating at all, because they had put the 'tempting' food *out of their mind*.

This was how my writing on weight control came into being and its foundation is that the ways in which you use your mind can make a major impact on the results you get. This book is your own personal guide to effective weight control and it uses some specialized approaches and techniques to help you bring about change, which I will be explaining as you move through the chapters. You will find a variety of ideas and suggestions for helping you achieve results and, if you follow the ideas through systematically, you will be able to make real progress.

As with any change process, you have to play an active part. This book will give you help, but ultimately it is up to you how well you do. If you are committed to making changes, the techiques presented here will show you how to achieve weight loss and give you help and support in achieving both short- and long-term goals.

Introduction: Starting Points

This section outlines the contents of the book and the benefits it will bring you.

Why read this book?

You will have your own personal reasons for reading a book such as this. You may simply have picked it off a shelf out of curiosity and found it intriguing; you may have decided it is time to make some changes and looked for help; or you may have spent a long time trying to manage your weight and found other sources of guidance did not help you achieve the results you really wanted.

Whatever your reasons, this book will help you in making changes you desire. It may be that you are concerned solely with your weight, or it might be that you wish to make bigger changes in your life and you realize that your weight is only a symptom, rather than the problem itself. The book will help, whichever of these is relevant to you; you can use it either simply to help you reduce weight, or as a foundation for enhancing your life overall.

Some of the ideas in this book may well be different from others you have come across. The approaches used are explained in chapter 2 and are based on well-established fields of study. The approach is that your experience is largely created by your mind. In other words, the way you think affects your interpretation of events and also influences the results you get in your life. Without thoughts there would be little or no development, creativity or progress – life depends on thinking.

Our thoughts, however, can lead us into negativity and unwanted consequences. So, if you can manage your thoughts effectively, you can start to get real results. The book will show you how to harness the power of thought in purposeful and powerful ways. In the past you may have had dreams about what you wanted; *Think Yourself Slim* will help you turn your wishes into reality.

What makes this book different?

The main theme in the book is that everyone is different and so any programme for achieving results needs to be tailored to you, as an individual. The book does not assume everyone is the same, but gives you individual and personal steps to take to ensure your success.

By following the book through, you will find out about several basic patterns of motivation and preference and begin to understand why something which works well for one person may be quite the wrong thing for another. By answering some of the questions asked in chapter 3, you will learn to identify your own personal motivational styles and then use this information in the design of your own personalized programme for controlling your weight.

What does the book contain?

To start with, the book has information on the power of your mind. As I have already said, your mind is a powerful instrument, which can produce for you either achievement or disappointment. You will find out, as you read, how your thoughts are made up of component parts, and you will find out how to change these parts in order to get the results you want.

You will also find some 'tests' in chapter 3. These tests are very simple, and have been designed to help you understand yourself better – an important factor in success. In particular, these tests will help you understand how you, personally, are motivated and how your motivation and preference patterns influence the ways in which you do things.

The book gives practical ideas and guidance on managing your weight and also on putting weight control in the context of your life as a whole. And finally, it gives you advice on healthy living and on finding out about useful resources and support networks.

It is *not* a diet book and it does not contain rules or fixed programmes of activity. Nor does it contain recipes, or an emphasis on calorie counting. It does, however, contain the basic principles which will enable you to make decisions about your life and how you want to lead it, especially what you want to do to control your weight.

How should you read and use this book?

The book is designed to be read in sequence, from start to finish, although, if you wish, you can skip some chapters or read some of the later ones earlier on. It is really important, however, to complete the self-assessment tests in chapter 3 before you move to the guidance given in chapters 4 and 5. This is because the processes will work better if you select the ones which fit best with the kind of person you are – and the tests will help you identify that. You will find some small illustrations in the margins in some chapters because in some cases I have suggested that you turn back to an earlier chapter and find a corresponding section with the same illustration, so that you can practise the techniques covered in more detail; this will become clear as you get to the relevant sections.

The book may be used alone, or together with any other programme you wish to combine it with. For example, if you feel you absolutely must follow a specific weight-control plan, you can use the book to help you do so, or if you want to take up a particular exercise regime, the book can help you keep to it. Each person has his or her own goals and preferences and you can use the book to help you follow whatever you choose to achieve results.

And finally . . .

The key to this book is self-understanding. Once you know your own patterns of thinking and behaving you can really make progress towards your goals. So, whatever your past experience is, make today the first day of your new approach to losing weight. It *is* possible to succeed in what you want to do because there are many things in your life which have been successes for you already. Maybe you cannot remember many things you have been successful in right now but, in later chapters, I will be showing you some simple ways of recalling successes. For now, the important thing is that you really want to commit yourself to starting a new programme which can result in you losing the weight you wish to.

So really decide that you can do it, *now*. Once you get started you will find it easier and easier to get results, as each small success will motivate you more to achieve the next one. As you read the book, imagine the sound of my voice encouraging you (I know we haven't met, but you can give me whatever voice you like in your imagination) and remember you have all the support you need to achieve your goals. Let's make a start together . . .

1
Weight: Fact and Fiction

> *This chapter explains the factors which are involved when people put on weight and discusses some common misconceptions about weight and weight control.*

Your personal history

When you were born you may have been a light baby or a heavy baby, but you would not have been 'overweight' at that time. Being overweight results from taking in more energy from your food than you can use up in day-to-day activity. So you have probably gained weight at some stage in your life and this may have been as a child, as an adolescent or as an adult (or a combination of all of these).

You may also have shared the experience of others, and found that your weight has cycled up and down at different periods; perhaps there were times when you were happy with your weight and times when you thought you weighed too much. This is a familiar situation for many people who 'diet', and we will be returning to the reasons for this later in the chapter.

So at present, you probably weigh more than you would like – possibly much more than you would like – and this may make itself obvious by your clothes being tight, your scales having higher readings and your mirror showing you a body you do not recognize as belonging to you. And you may have decided it is time to do something about it.

How you can tell whether you need to lose weight and, if you do, how much

How do you tell how much weight you need to lose? Perhaps you think you should go by what you weighed at a particular time in your life; perhaps when you left school or when you got married. Perhaps you have an 'ideal' weight in mind; maybe a weight you have been at one time, or maybe a weight which you just think would be right for you. Or maybe you just want to weigh 'less', without being too clear about what weight this would be exactly.

There are some ways of telling what your 'ideal' weight is likely to be and I would like to tell you about these before we move on.

Let's start with how to know if you are overweight. A simple way is by using what is known as the 'pinch test'. This is very simple; you just go to different parts of your body and try to take hold of some flesh between your thumb and first finger. If you can grip more than 1in/2.5mm thickness of flesh in this way, you may well be carrying too much fat. Remember, though, that fat in certain parts of the body affects you differently and you can read more about this in the Appendix.

Another way is to check how your clothes fit. If you are an adult and have taken a particular size in clothes for some time, and now find they are becoming tight on you, you may well be carrying more weight than is right for you. A third way is to compare your present weight with the 'average' weights of people of the same sex and height as you and see if you are within 'normal' boundaries. You will find how to do this in the Appendix, but again remember that 'average' weights are only a *guide,* not an absolute rule.

It may also be that you have been told by your doctor that you need to lose weight for health reasons. So you need to check, before starting a programme, whether you need to lose weight at all and, if so, how much. It is also important to check whether there are any reasons why you should not lose weight at this time. For example, if you are pregnant, if you have not reached adulthood and are still growing, or if you have a medical complaint which could be adversely affected by restricting your food intake or by exercising more, you should make sure you see your doctor and get confirmation before starting.

Assuming there are no medical reasons to prevent you from beginning a programme, you will probably benefit from losing weight if:

- your doctor has told you to lose weight
- the 'pinch test' shows more than 1in/2.5mm of fat at several places on your body
- your clothes have rapidly become very tight on you and there is no medical reason for this
- your body fat percentage is above the recommended level (*see* Appendix)
- your weight-to-height ratio is above the recommended average (*see* Appendix)

And remember, losing weight should be a gradual process. If you try to slim down too quickly, your body will simply think it is being starved and start using food more economically. In the long term, a slow and steady reduction will be much more effective and result in permanent weight loss, not simply a temporary loss with subsequent regain.

What about cellulite?

There is still disagreement about the term 'cellulite'. It is sometimes used to describe what often appears as lumpy or dimpled areas on the body, where fat under the skin seems to have turned into unsightly masses. Some doctors do not accept that cellulite exists as a separate kind of fatty tissue, whereas others (and more or less all of those working in, and writing about, the 'beauty' industry) use the term as an accepted fact.

People who believe that cellulite exists say that it can be reduced through massage, drinking plenty of fluid to flush toxins out of the body, eating a healthy diet and taking exercise. These are just the things which are recommended in any general weight-loss programme so, if you follow these principles, you will improve your weight and appearance, whatever name you give to your fat!

Why do people become overweight?

Weight is put on when food intake exceeds energy output; this is a simple fact. If you eat food you do not need – for example, if you eat when you are not hungry – the consequence will probably be that food is stored as fat.

There are a few people who have medical conditions which make their bodies poor at managing the food resources supplied to them. In general, however, excess weight only results from eating too much and exercising too little. As other writers have pointed out, obesity tends not to be found in countries where there is a famine; it is a symptom of access to plentiful supplies of food. To say that excess weight comes from eating too much does not tackle the underlying causes, however. People eat for a variety of reasons, quite apart from hunger.

Why might you eat when you do not need the food? The first three reasons we will be considering are:

- not paying attention
- developing habits
- being influenced by your 'unconscious mind'

Let us take each of these in turn.

Not paying attention

First, you may actually have no underlying 'problem' but simply have gained weight without being too aware of it. One reason for this happening could be that you have simply been gradually increasing your daily intake by small amounts which, over the months and years, add up to weight gain. This can happen very easily if you do not monitor what you eat, or if you are not careful about eating healthily and make a habit of snacking on high-calorie foods.

Developing habits

Alternatively, you may simply have been eating out of habit, rather than waiting until you are hungry before having a meal. Habits are easy things to get into and the good news is that, if you have developed one habit, it means you have the general capability of forming habits and can therefore learn new, healthier, ones quite easily.

Some situations in which people eat out of habit are:

- watching television
- driving
- sitting at a computer

I am sure you can add other situations of your own to this list.

You will know if you frequently eat just because the food is there, or because you have become used to nibbling in certain places or at certain times. This awareness and recognition is a good step on the way to achieving control of when and where you eat.

Being influenced by your 'unconscious' mind

You may not have realized that your mind works in quite complex ways. It is generally held that two kinds of process can go on in your mind. The first is what we call 'conscious' processa, which means that you are aware of the thoughts in your mind as they occur, for example seeing a cream bun and *knowing* that you are being tempted by it.

The second kind of process is called 'unconscious' and means that you may do things without a completely conscious awareness of what you are doing, or why you are doing it. So you might find yourself half-way through a packet of biscuits without realizing you had eaten so many (not knowing *what* you were doing), or you could find yourself putting a high-calorie snack food in your trolley at the supermarket without remembering that that particular brand had featured in a TV advertisement the evening before (not knowing *why* you are doing something).

We all have things which affect our behaviour and

which are not always readily accessible to our conscious mind. For example, you may have been told off by someone as a child and now react to people speaking in a similar tone of voice without knowing why. What has happened is that a past experience (or sometimes an anticipated future experience) influences your behaviour without you knowing it is doing so. It is useful to know that your mind can work in this way, because eating habits often stem from factors which are out of our conscious awareness and, if you can understand how and why you do particular things, they often become much easier to control or change.

Now let us move on to some of the other reasons why people eat when they are not hungry. I shall be talking about five of these in this section.

- eating because of your emotions
- eating as a displacement activity or substitution for something else
- eating as an excuse
- eating as self-punishment
- eating as a way of being able to control some part of your life

Let us take each of these categories in turn and find out more about them.

Eating because of your emotions

See if any of the following might apply to you:

- I eat because I am bored.
- I eat because I am unhappy.
- I eat because I feel under pressure at work or in other areas of my life.

- I eat because I feel other people expect me to do so.
- I eat because I feel bad if food is wasted.

If you have answered 'Yes' to any of these, you are not alone. Often eating is not related solely to hunger, but results from compensation for other factors, such as feeling bad or having too much to do. Often such eating is not done at an entirely conscious level, so you may find yourself eating without really wishing to. I will be talking more about this later in the chapter.

Eating as a displacement or substitution activity

For some people, eating is what we call a displacement activity: something they do as a substitute for something else. Very often this is called 'comfort eating'.

See if any of the following apply to you:

- I eat instead of smoking.
- I eat because I do not have any work to do.
- I eat because I do not get affection from anyone or have any friends.
- I eat instead of resting or sleeping.

Sometimes you may know you are eating as a substitute, for example putting food into your mouth instead of reaching for a cigarette. At other times, however, the substitution may not have reached your conscious mind. Take tiredness, for example. Many people find they eat when they are tired and do not realize they are not actually hungry. Having a sleep is what their body really needs but, because they are not able to sleep at the time, they may interpret the tiredness signals as hunger.

So being able to know what signals your body is giving you, so that you can tell if you are actually hungry or not, is really important when managing your weight.

Eating as an excuse

For some people, food is an excuse. For example, you might not want to get into a permanent relationship with another person. This might be because you have previously had a bad experience, because you are afraid of the commitment, or for other reasons. In a situation like this, people react differently. One person might simply say that they are not ready to have a close relationship. Another person might make an excuse, such as being too busy, or having to care for children or elderly relatives.

Some people, however, do not make a direct excuse, but behave in such a way that their relationship is affected. This can be a conscious process, where they may think that if they weigh a lot they will become unattractive to others and so, by overeating, they literally put up a physical barrier to personal contact. And sometimes it may be unconscious, so that a person is not aware of the fact that he is overeating in order to avoid contact with others. In some of these cases, once the person becomes aware that his eating is having this result, he is able to face the issue head on and either finds ways of telling the other person directly that he does not want to be with her or, better still, helps himself to become better able to handle relationships. In many of these cases the person's weight then becomes more 'normal' as he tackles the issues in his life which have given rise to the weight gain.

If this sounds like you, you will find that, by bringing this process into your conscious awareness, you can help yourself decide what your attitudes and feelings are towards relationships. Once you know that you are avoiding relationships, you can decide whether this is appropriate behaviour or not. It may be just that, in the past, you did not know how to handle relationships, but you are now much better able to do so. It may be much easier now for you to accept that you can have a successful and rewarding relationship with someone else and not have to overeat in order to avoid this.

Eating as self-punishment

In some cases, eating may be a punishment. Some people really feel they do not deserve to be attractive, successful or loved. If this is so, they may put on weight to justify their belief that they are unworthy or 'bad'.

What they are doing is punishing themselves for being who they are. The real problem is not the weight, it is their attitude to themselves; their 'self-image' or level of self-esteem. If this is the case, it is important to tackle this underlying issue as well as embarking on the weight-control programme for, if it is not dealt with, they are likely to continue to sabotage their efforts to change.

Eating as a way of controlling part of your life

Finally, it can happen that people overeat when they feel they are not in control of their lives. This is common in serious food disorders such as anorexia and bulimia. The people concerned do not always realize that this is what is happening, but it is likely that they either starve themselves, or overeat and then vomit up their food, in order to gain some control over at least one area of their lives. People who do this are often affecting not only themselves, but others close to them also, and the effects of their eating processes can have major consequences, not only for their own health but for the functioning of their wider family.

Why do some people find it easier to keep to weight-control programmes?

You may feel that it is much easier for some people to control their weight than for others. If you think you are a person who finds controlling your weight difficult, there could be a number of reasons you give for this.

The first reason could be that you are easily tempted by appetizing food. The fact is, though, that lots of people are tempted, and those who have ways of dealing with temptation tend to be more successful. So I will be giving you ways of countering temptation in chapters 5 and 7.

The second reason may be that you have a medical condition which makes it difficult for you to lose weight. Although this is possible, it does not apply to the majority of people who are overweight. If you really believe this is the case, you should consult your doctor for advice on weight control but, unless your medical condition is exceptional, there is likely to be a good deal you can do to reduce weight through healthy eating and exercise plans.

The third reason could be that you are genetically predisposed to putting on weight. This is often used by people as an excuse for being overweight, 'Oh,' they say, 'I cannot help it – all my family are large.' There can be an element of truth in this, although it is seldom the only reason for not losing weight, so let us see why people can vary in their susceptibility to putting on weight.

There is a range of 'body types' which can react differently to weight management; see if you can recognize yourself in one of them. The three main types are

11

called ectomorphs, mesomorphs and endomorphs. Put simply, ectomorphs are people who are naturally thin, often with angular features and long bones. This is a typical shape for long-distance runners, for example. Mesomorphs are naturally muscular and look athletic; sprinters are good examples. And endomorphs have more rounded features, often with a higher percentage of body fat – sumo wrestlers, possibly!

Most people tend towards a combination of two of these types and, the closer you are to one of them, the more difficult you may find it to adjust your weight. So the naturally slim ectomorphs can find it difficult to put on muscle, while the naturally rounded endomorphs may struggle if they need to slim down, even with regular diet and exercise.

The reasons for having one or other body type stem from your genetic make-up, an important part of which produces your muscle cells. There are two major types of muscle fibre in your body, known as 'fast twitch' and 'slow twitch'. We have, on average, 50 per cent of each in our bodies, and we cannot change one type to another. Fast-twitch muscle fibres are quick to react but can tire easily, and slow-twitch muscle fibres are slow to react but resistant to fatigue. Slow-twitch muscle fibres are those which prefer working aerobically (see chapter 8) and fast-twitch muscle fibres generally prefer working anaerobically, although some can also work aerobically as well. If you have a high proportion of slow-twitch muscles, you will react better to aerobic exercise; the kind of exercises which raise your pulse rate and make your metabolism work faster, burning off fat more effectively. If you have a very high percentage of fast-twitch muscles, you may struggle to do aerobic exercises and be better suited to the more 'explosive', anaerobic exercises instead. Unfortunately, you cannot check your own balance of fast- and slow-twitch muscles, but you do have a uniquely personal distribution of these muscle fibres and your ability to alter your weight or muscle distribution will be based, in part, on this balance.

And do remember that, although you may be predisposed to having a higher proportion of one or other muscle fibre type, it is actually very rare for a person not to respond at all to good diet and exercise. So being aware of your natural body type is useful, but you should not use it as an excuse for failing to lose weight in your programme. And remember that, even if genetics plays a large part in predisposing people to weight gains, it is interesting to note that statistics show that people now are generally heavier than they were ten years ago, yet their genes are the same as they were then, so genetics alone cannot possibly take all the blame!

Why don't people stick to weight-control programmes, when they know they should be doing so?

To understand this, you need to know a bit about psychology. Put very simply, people do things for a wide variety of reasons, some to do with their personal resources and abilities and some to do with their responses to external situations.

I will be going into individual motivation patterns in chapter 3; the main thing you need to know here is that it is not just as simple as knowing you *should* be doing something. If you take as an example a person who has agoraphobia, it is no use telling her to pull herself together and go out – if she could, she would. There are things in her mind which prevent her from doing what she would like to do and, until she tackles the mental as well as the physical elements, she may find it hard to make changes.

One particular factor which is influential in the success of a personal programme is what is often called 'secondary gain'. This means that there are things you gain from staying as you are rather than making changes, and you may or may not be aware of these secondary gains at a conscious level. Let us take the example of agoraphobia again. You might say there are no gains in this, but a person who is agoraphobic prob-ably has visitors and people who do things for him. Of course he is not 'choosing' to be agoraphobic but, at an unconscious level, he may fear that he will not have any friends or support if he becomes 'better'. So his unconscious mind keeps him dependent on others, even though, consciously, he may be very upset about his behaviour.

This is an extreme example, but just apply the same principle to yourself. Do you enjoy going out with friends for meals? If so, the social aspect of eating may be your secondary gain; if you stopped going to restaur-ants, you would deprive yourself of company, as well as reducing your food intake. If you devote a bit of thought to this, you will probably be able to find things you would miss if you changed your eating and exercise patterns. Thinking these things out before you start a programme is vital, otherwise your unconscious mind may well sabotage your efforts. I will be coming back to this topic later in the book.

Another reason why people do not always persist with weight-control programmes is that they sometimes reach a 'plateau', where they seem to stop losing weight. It is possible to become disillusioned at this point and think of giving up. But it is important to remember that it is a common stage to go through and is simply your body readjusting to its new intake levels. It is only a temporary phase and, once it has passed, you can continue losing weight until you reach your target.

This part of the chapter has discussed some of the reasons why people overeat and have difficulty changing their behaviour. Some of these may sound familiar to you and others may surprise you but, if you do recognize yourself in any of these patterns, you will have gained some useful information which we will be taking further in the chapters which follow. Let's move on now to consider some common misconceptions about food and weight control.

Some myths and rumours about losing weight

The following sections present some popularly held views. Although there is much evidence that they are untrue, people continue to believe them. Sometimes this belief is reinforced by companies selling products aimed at people who wish to lose weight. The weight-control industry is so large, and generates so much money, that it has a vested interest in people continuing to believe some things which are now recognized as untrue or, worse still, counterproductive.

Here are some of the myths surrounding weight control.

Dieting works

For years, a 'diet' was the acceptable way to lose weight. You embarked on a programme of calorie-counting and restriction in the hope of losing excess weight on a permanent basis. Unfortunately, such diets generally resulted, at best, in temporary weight loss, with subsequent regain. The reason for this is that these diets did not educate their users in good eating patterns and, once the diet was ended, the previous pattern of less healthy eating was generally resumed. In most cases all the weight lost was put back, and often more besides.

Very low-calorie diets work

These diets rely on excessively low calorie intakes. They do work in the short term, because your body is simply getting insufficient sustenance to maintain current weight and also because they cause substantial water loss which, in itself, shows a lower weight on your scales. The problem is that, once your body gets used to a lower basic intake, it can adjust its metabolism accordingly. Once you come off the diet, your basic daily requirement for food has dropped and, if you go back to a more normal daily intake, you will probably gain weight again at an even faster rate than before.

Miracle pills exist

There are many pills, diet bars, drinks and other products designed to substitute for food, to reduce your desire for food or, increasingly nowadays, to prevent certain foods (generally saturated fats – *see* chapter 8) from being absorbed by your body. Even when such products do what is claimed for them, there can be drawbacks. They are introducing substances into your body which may produce side-effects and there are recorded instances of serious health problems arising from some such products (although others, of course, will have a good record of testing and safety). Medical supervision is advisable and, again, even if they work, these products do not educate you to a healthier eating programme, which means that weight is likely to creep on again.

Everyone can look like a supermodel

As I explained earlier, everyone is different. Your basic height and body proportions are fixed by the time you are an adult. Some people have long arms and legs; some have angular faces; some have short necks; some have large feet; some have small hips. You cannot change these basic proportions. What you can do with weight control is to make the most of, and enhance, your own proportions; what you *cannot* do is become someone else, however hard you may try.

Will-power is the most important thing

Will-power is not a commodity, something that some people have and others do not. It is a mental process which, like other mental processes, can be developed. But will-power in itself is not what makes people succeed; it is the real *desire* to achieve a goal and *knowing how* to work towards it that counts. All the will-power in the world will not help if you do not know what to apply the will-power to.

Exercise is hard work

When you are not keeping absolutely immobile you are exercising. Just walking from room to room, putting on your clothes and eating a meal are forms of exercise.

17

What people generally mean, if they say they think exercise is hard work, is that the forms of exercise which have been suggested to them are ones they do not want to do. Once you find the right kind of exercise for you, you will really be able to enjoy it.

Weight loss in itself means fat loss

This is not true, because muscle tissues weigh more than fat. So you may increase weight and still be fitter, as you have a greater muscle-to-fat ratio than before, or you may lose weight and be less fit because you have accumulated fat and lost muscle fibre. This is one reason why weighing yourself is not necessarily the best way to assess your fitness levels; checking whether your clothes are getting looser, whether you are looking more toned and whether you have more energy is probably a better assessment.

You can look exactly as you did 10, 20 or 30 years ago

Nobody can turn the clock back. Although everyone can look their best for their age, certain physiological changes inevitably accompany the ageing process. For example, your skin loses some of its elasticity and is likely to wrinkle, especially if you sunbathe a good deal. Muscle mass tends to diminish with age and hair and skin colour fades. So you can certainly improve your weight and your general appearance, but you cannot achieve miracles.

Stopping smoking makes you put on weight

This is a commonly held belief, as some people do seem to put on weight (often around the stomach, which has particular health risks associated with it – *see* Appendix) when they stop smoking. There are a number of possible reasons for this. First, your taste buds improve, so food tastes better and you may want to eat more of it. It also appears that nicotine increases the rate at which your body burns off excess food, so you can gain a few pounds temporarily after quitting smoking. This tends to be only a small increase and is unlikely to have much of an effect except with very heavy smokers. It is also likely that blood sugar levels remain higher when nicotine is in the body, because of its effect on insulin metabolism. And there are major health implications, such as the risk of lung cancer, arising from the habit of smoking.

The most likely result of stopping smoking is a need to have a substitute activity; something to do with your hands, or to put in your mouth, instead. So if you work out in advance what to do to occupy yourself after you do stop smoking, and if you have a sensible programme of healthy eating and exercise, it is unlikely that you will gain any weight.

Medical treatments can substitute for sensible eating and exercise

There are many forms of treatment now available, generally through the private medical market, which aim to help people reduce their weight. Although these can be effective, they are generally a remedy for extreme obesity rather than a practical approach to everyday weight control. And they do not re-educate your body, so you can still regain weight after using such treatments. Some treatments now available include:

- **Liposuction.** This is a process whereby certain chemicals are introduced into the body which dissolve fat; the dissolved fat is then pumped out. This does reduce volume and weight, but can also leave loose and wrinkled skin and an uneven surface appearance, and there may be side-effects resulting from the chemicals used. In addition, people undergoing this treatment often have to wear tight bandages for several weeks until their body has taken on a new shape. Of course the treatment costs money too; it is expensive.

- **Tummy tucks.** This is where fat is surgically removed from certain areas, often the stomach, although other operations can involve breast reduction and treatment of other parts of the body. This is a major surgical procedure, carrying the risks of any major operation. It can also be painful and take time to recover from. Again, it is an expensive procedure.

- **Teeth wiring.** This is a process whereby a person's teeth are temporarily wired together so that he can only take in liquids and is unable to eat solid food. Generally this has to result in weight loss, but is uncomfortable and unsightly and does not re-educate you to healthy eating patterns.

- **Stomach stapling.** This is an even more extreme process, which involves an operation to staple together part of the stomach so that it is uncomfortable to eat more than an extremely small amount of food without feelings of discomfort. A similar, newer, procedure, is to insert a balloon into the stomach, which is then inflated, also creating the feeling of being very full. These are major operations with accompanying risks. Again, they do not re-educate anyone to better eating and exercising patterns.

Although most people working in cosmetic surgery are reputable, there are some who are not, or who are less experienced, and there can be no guarantee of the success of such operations as I have described.

Non-medical treatments make a major difference

There are many things you can do to assist a weight-control programme. Many facilities are available at leisure centres, spas and beauty salons, which are certainly aids to managing your weight. Although these treatments can help, they are not a substitute for food control and active exercise. Some of these treatments are:

- **Saunas and Turkish baths.** These involve sitting in heated rooms either with steam (Turkish) or in dry heat (sauna). Although they are enjoyable, any weight loss is simply water lost through sweating and it will quickly be replaced as soon as you take a drink.
- **Wraps.** This involves bandaging the body with cloths, often infused with herbal products or clays. Again, sweating is caused and impurities removed; weight loss is still likely to be very temporary, resulting from water loss, although often an immediate, short-lasting reduction in specific places can be obtained.
- **Toning tables.** This involves lying or sitting on a table which moves, and you resist its movement with different parts of your body. Toning tables can be helpful, but doing similar exercises in a gym or exercise class will probably burn off many more calories. Unless these tables are supervised by experienced staff, with good knowledge of physiology, you will really need to know your own body well, and what movements are safe for you to do, so that you can be

21

confident in asking for the movement of the table to be stopped if you feel you are being taken out of a reasonable comfort zone.

Hypnotherapy and similar treatments work all on their own, without you having to do anything

This might possibly be true in some cases, but generally you still have to put in some effort. Hypnotic suggestions are really helpful in a weight-loss programme, but you still have to buy and cook the right foods and take the exercise. Self-hypnosis is also a useful aid to weight control but, again, you still need a practical programme to accompany it.

Only certain people can be successful

This is a real myth. Everyone is successful at something, even if they sometimes do not recognize the fact. Once you know how, you can be really successful at managing yourself; you just need to learn the techniques and then apply them.

Because you have not succeeded in the past, you cannot be successful in the future

This is a wonderful way of ensuring you do not achieve your goals. The past is just that – the past. The future is something new. In the past you had baby teeth, did not know how to tie shoelaces and had not yet learned the language you speak. And now you have changed all those things. Living is a process of change and development and, just as you learned a language, so you can learn how to control your weight. Past 'failures' are not predictors of the future, they are simply lessons in what to avoid next time round.

Once you have lost weight, that is all you have to do

Weight loss is just the beginning. If you really want to make changes in your weight, you have to be prepared to continue the process and *maintain* your weight loss. This means continuing with a healthy eating and exercising programme – for the rest of your life! Unless you are prepared to do this, your weight gain will probably only be temporary.

This chapter has given you some answers to the questions you may have had about weight control. You might have other questions; if so, later chapters cover many further aspects which will give you both information and guidance.

In the next chapter, some of the specific approaches used in the book are described.

2
Aids to Change

*The first part of this chapter introduces you
to two approaches to enhancing personal
effectiveness: Neuro-Linguistic Programming
and Accelerated Learning. It then outlines the
major elements involved in achievement and
describes the process you will be following in
later chapters in order to bring about the
changes you wish for. The second part of the
chapter introduces you to a range of techniques
which can help you achieve results. The
techniques are mainly to do with thought
processes and will give you ways of using your
mind flexibly and effectively.*

APPROACHES TO PERSONAL EFFECTIVENESS

Neuro-LInguistic Programming (NLP)

NLP is an approach to personal effectiveness which grew
out of the work of a group of people based at the
University of California in the early 1970s. In turn, their
work was grounded in earlier thinking, in some cases
going back centuries. NLP offers ways of bringing about
personal change through modifying your ways of thinking, feeling and behaving.

NLP arose from the study of how people who were
really good at what they did got their results. Once you
know what makes someone effective, you can use her
ways of doing things to improve your own effectiveness.

This does not mean you have to become exactly like that person, it simply means copying a little of what she does in order to achieve results.

This is exactly the process children use when they learn; they watch someone else doing something, or listen to how someone says something, and then they copy it. Of course, this does mean that sometimes they get it 'wrong' as they copy what they think they have seen, or they copy what they think is appropriate in a particular situation. In order to be successful, it is important to know that what you are copying is appropriate and useful and to be able to copy it correctly.

NLP helps you copy things well, so that you can improve your results. A large part of this book is about the process of doing things differently, and you will find suggestions for ways of changing how you think and what you do so that you can achieve more.

Accelerated Learning

Accelerated Learning is recognizing how you, personally, learn. As the term implies, learning can be made quicker if certain steps are taken and, through Accelerated Learning, you can identify your preferred ways of learning and create environments where you can learn enjoyably and easily.

One of the principles of Accelerated Learning is that environments are really important. In other words, we are influenced by the place we are in and what is happening in it. For example, if you want to exercise at home, but you do not have a space which is inviting, you may not bother. If everything is cluttered, noisy and draughty, it may be really hard to get down to exercising in an enthusiastic way. By making your environment more welcoming and pleasant, you improve your chances of success.

Accelerated Learning also emphasizes that people's own motivational and preference patterns are vitally important in their learning. By understanding what 'turns you on' you will be better able to start, and continue, any programme you choose. In the next chapter I will show you how to identify your own patterns, and use the knowledge of them in designing and following your weight-control programme.

The five major elements of achievement

There are various factors which contribute to successful goal achievement; David Gordon and Graham Dawes, well-known NLP trainers, generally consider five as being basic to effectiveness. The five main elements of success are:

- having appropriate, measurable and achievable **goals**
- having the **behavioural skills** that the situation requires
- having positive and motivating **thoughts**
- having resourceful and supportive **feelings**
- having **beliefs** which make it possible to progress and move forward

These different elements work together as a total system to produce your results. If you have clear goals, think positively and feel resourceful, have the skills to do what you need and believe that you can succeed, you are more likely to achieve results. The opposite is true too; if you are hazy about what you want, have negative thoughts and feelings, lack the knowledge and techniques to follow a suitable programme and believe you will be unsuccessful, you are less likely to succeed.

So working on each of these areas is an important factor in success. In this book, we will be covering each of them and I will be showing you how to make the most of your own abilities. And, by the way, as well as using this process for weight control, you can also use it in any other area of your life where you have a goal you would like to achieve, or where you would like to make changes in the ways in which you think, feel and behave.

The process you will be following in this book

This book takes you through a simple and straight-forward three-part process. The first part involves identifying what you do at present (your **present state**). The second part involves considering what you want instead of what you have at present (your **desired state**). The third part involves working out what steps you need to take to move from your present situation to your desired situation (**steps to take**).

We will be following this three-part process because it will make it easy for you to understand the gap between where you are now and where you want to be and the ideas presented throughout the book will give you practical ways of taking the steps required to be successful.

THE FOUNDATIONS OF SUCCESS

This section will show you some things about how your mind works. It will take you through a series of exercises designed to give you greater mental flexibility. This is important, because how you *think* has a major effect on how you *feel* and on how you *behave*. Once you get your mind working effectively you will be well on the way to succeeding.

The exercises will give you some unusual ways of thinking. You will probably find some of them very easy to do and others may be more of a challenge. It is well worth taking the time to practise because you will be needing these skills when you come to chapter 4, which will give you practical steps to take to make the changes you desire.

Each of the sections which follows has a small illustration. The illustrations include an eye (for visualizing), an ear (for hearing) and so on. Again, when you come to chapter 4, you will find the same symbols appearing. When you see a symbol in chapter 4, you should return to the section in this chapter with the same symbol and reread the exercises. This will help you a good deal, especially with the activities which require changes in thinking.

How your mind produces thoughts

Leaving aside the question of 'extrasensory' processes such as thought transference, your awareness derives from the use of your different senses: sight, hearing, taste, smell and touch. These senses, produced by your brain, in conjunction with other physiological processes in your body, generate both mental and physical sensations.

The physical sensations are generally obvious enough; you know when you can see something or hear something; you know when you feel hot or cold, or energetic or tired; you know when something tastes good or bad. But there is a mental component to sensing, too, and you may not always be so aware of the detail of this kind of process.

For example, if you were asked to remember a recent event, such as a journey, a holiday, a meal in a restaurant or a visit to the theatre, you would use a wide range of mental processes to recall the event. For many of us, however, these mental processes are out of conscious awareness and we simply say: 'I remember that.' Similarly, if you were asked to imagine something you have not actually experienced, for example a trip to the moon, flying like a bird or being presented with a Nobel Prize, you would also go through a range of mental processes to imagine the occurrence, but you would probably simply say: 'Yes, I can imagine that' (or maybe, 'No, I cannot imagine that').

What your mind is actually doing while this process is going on is presenting you with 'internal representations' of your different senses. So, your mind might be making pictures (visualizing), producing imaginary sounds, tastes and smells, making you aware of tactile sensations or giving you a sense of emotional feelings.

The fascinating thing about all of this is that our minds are not good at separating fact and fiction. Of course we 'know' when something is not real, but if you imagine a slice of lemon in your mouth it may begin to water, or if you think of a sad event you may feel like crying. These events are not 'real' in the 'here and now', they are simply memories or imaginations, yet your mind treats them *as if* they were real.

What we are about to do is to make the most of your mind's ability to treat things you present it as if they

29

were real. We shall work through a range of exercises, designed to give you more flexibility in how you think, and to show you that you can be more in control of both your mind and your physical responses than you might have imagined. Let us take these processes one at a time.

Picturing things in your mind

Picturing things in your mind (visualizing) is an important element in thinking. How often do you picture how things will go before they happen? Equally, how often do you play back in your head an event which has already taken place? In this section I will show you how to create and manipulate, images in your mind.

So, to begin, picture the following objects: a house, a car, a tree, an aeroplane, a camera, a horse, a telephone, a guitar, a magazine and an apple.

Now take one of these objects, say the tree, and imagine it very, very small and then very, very large. Imagine it close to you and then far away. Imagine it quite still, as if in a photograph, and then with its branches and leaves moving, as if in the wind. Now imagine the tree being yellow, then purple, then white, as if covered with snow. Now picture the tree very clearly, in sharp focus, and then looking rather fuzzy or hazy, as if you were seeing it in fog or through a film of water. Now imagine the tree has fruit on it. Now imagine it has shoes hanging from the branches. Now imagine it has a small door in its trunk and the door is open and you can see a tiny person standing at the entrance.

Once you have been successful in doing this exercise,

you will have seen how your mind has the capability of producing a wide range of images. If you found the exercise hard to do, you can practise visualization skills by doing the following:

- Look in a mirror, describe to yourself the detail of how your face looks. Now close your eyes and remember those same details.
- Open a magazine or book, look at an illustration, again describe to yourself what you see, then close your eyes and remember the images.

By practising these techniques you will become more skilled at visualizing and internal focusing and this will help considerably with some of the processes for achieving results which I will be describing later in the book. And, by the way, if you are one of those people who find it really hard to visualize, you can do other things instead, as you will find out below.

Creating imaginary sounds

As well as pictures, our minds can produce sounds. In this section we will go through some exercises you can do to develop your ability to imagine sounds in your head.

Imagine a bird singing, an express train going through a tunnel, the sound of waves breaking on a beach, a jet plane overhead, rain, a piano being played, footsteps on a wooden floor and a cricket ball being hit by a bat. Now, in your head, hear yourself counting from one to ten.

Now take the footsteps on the wooden floor. Hear them very loud, as if they are getting close to you; now

31

hear them quietly, as if going off into the distance. Now imagine the sounds of the steps as if they are coming from your left and now from your right. Now imagine the feet have bells round the ankles and think how the footsteps would sound with bare feet and ankle bells. Now imagine the wooden floor has changed to wet tiles and imagine how bare feet would sound on the wet floor. Now imagine there are many more footsteps – several people – and notice how that would sound. Finally, imagine how the footsteps would sound if they were made by a bird on the wooden floor.

Doing these exercises will help you tune into the different ways your mind can represent sounds and this will be very helpful in the processes we will be following later.

Experimenting with 'self-talk' or the conversations you may have with yourself in your head

You may well be familiar with this process, which is a part of your sense of hearing. Self-talk is the little voice in your head which tells you how things are going. If you have ever had difficulty in getting to sleep at nights, it may well be self-talk which kept you awake.

Sometimes self-talk is very positive and encouraging, but at other times it can be negative and destructive. Once you know how to control your inner voices, you will be better equipped to give yourself positive messages about the future and what you want to achieve in it. So have a go at the following exercises:

Say something to yourself, in your head, about the place you are in right now. For example, if it is a room, you might comment on how it is furnished and decorated; if it is a garden, you might tell yourself about the kinds of plants, the colour of the sky and any sounds you can hear around you. As you do this, notice how loud or quiet your voice seems. Notice the tone of voice you 'hear'. Notice how quickly or slowly your voice seems to be speaking.

Now, in your mind, make your voice sound louder, then higher, then deeper, then softer, then faster, then slower. Make your voice sound serious, then humorous (perhaps like a cartoon voice).

Now hear your voice saying something very nice about you. Now hear it saying something very encouraging about your ability to achieve your goals.

Working with internal voices is a good start to making changes in your personal life. Often, we are prevented from changing by 'telling ourselves' that we will not succeed, that things will be hard or that other people will not like us if we change. Changing such self-talk can overcome negative thinking and put you on the road to success.

Using your mind to imagine smells and tastes

Just as your mind can produce pictures and sounds, it can also produce imaginary smells and tastes. Have a go at the following to develop your mental powers in these areas.

Imagine the scent of a rose, the aroma of floor polish, the smell of a swimming pool. Now imagine how a rose would smell if it had been dipped in paint, or if it had been sprayed with lemon juice.

Now imagine the taste of an apple, of orange juice

and of strong mints. Now imagine how a banana tastes when it is under-ripe, over-ripe and just right.

Doing these exercises stimulates your brain to create imaginary experiences for you, a process which we will be returning to in later chapters.

Imagining how things feel to your touch

In the previous exercises, you practised imagining or remembering sights, sounds, smells and tastes; in this part you will be creating tactile (sense of touch) experiences.

Imagine how a piece of velvet feels when you touch it; how your shoes feel when you put them on; what it feels like to lie in warm water and then in cool water; how it feels to sit in a comfortable chair; how it feels to sit in the sunshine; how it feels when you hold someone's hand. Now imagine what it would feel like if your hair was very long and rested on your shoulders; how it would feel if you could fly through the air like a bird; how it would feel if you were able to run as fast as a gazelle.

Producing and changing emotional feelings

Now let us turn to emotions. For these exercises you will need to think about some past experiences, so find a relaxing place where you will not be disturbed, take your time to get comfortable and then start the exercises.

Remember a time when you felt really excited about something and notice what that feeling is composed of. For example do you have a particular sensation in your

34

head or your stomach? Are you breathing at a particular speed? Does your face have a particular expression? Are you sitting or standing in a particular position? Now remember a time when you felt very relaxed. Again, as you recall that time, notice how you are breathing, what sensations you have in your body and whether you are keeping still or shifting position. Now think about a time when you felt very confident about something. Again notice how this brings about changes in your body. Finally, think about a time when you felt very motivated to do something and, again, notice what sensations and movements accompany that feeling. Become aware of how your body changes with the different emotions and notice the differences in your posture, movement, breathing, expression, and internal sensations as you change from one emotion to another.

Being able to change your feelings is an excellent skill. Many people think they are at the mercy of their emotions and that external events control them. They say things like: 'Oh, that person *made me* really angry', or 'I just *have to* get upset when I think of people dying from incurable diseases'. In fact, nobody 'makes' you angry; they just do things which you then react to. And you do not 'have' to be upset by anything; of course you may have a tendency to let things upset you, but you can be far more in control of your feelings than you may have thought. And, if you control your feelings, you may also be able to think of ways of helping situations, which would be impossible if you reacted simply out of emotion.

By doing exercises in which you remember certain feelings, you will realize that your body does different things when you are in positive or negative moods. Knowing this is the first step to being in control of your emotions. If you really want to *feel* different, you can put your body into the posture for the feeling you want, you can get your breathing into the rhythm and depth you want and you can allow your face to have on it the expression you want. You will find this actually creates the feeling you wish for, and having good feelings is one key to success with weight control. When you can feel good just by choosing to do so, you are less likely to turn to food for comfort.

Seeing things from another point of view

We all perceive things from our own perspective or point of view. It is important to do this, because self-preservation is vital to personal survival. However, as we live in a society with other people, it is also important to be able to see things from other people's points of view if we are to relate to them well. It is very useful to be able to take on other perspectives when working towards weight control (or other similar personal life changes) because single-minded perspectives often blinker our vision and stop us seeing how things could be different.

In the following exercises, I will take you through some ways of shifting perspective.

When you are next in a train (or on a bus or in a restaurant), look at a fellow passenger or diner. Imagine you are in that person's seat and think how the train carriage or dining area would look to you if you were in his position. Now, still imagining you are in his seat, think what it would be like if you looked towards yourself from that position. How do you think you might look to someone sitting over there?

Think back to a conversation you had with someone, when you both had very different views of a situation. Remember what you said to her and what she said to you. Now imagine you are that other person and, in your mind, imagine yourself saying what she said; really *feel* yourself saying those things. Does this experience make you feel any differently about what the other person said? Think about what might have happened to you in your life to produce your views and about how those particular life experiences might have resulted in your becoming different as a person.

Choose a person who is a very different shape and size from you. He can either be someone you actually meet face to face, or someone you see on TV. Observe him moving around and notice how he stands, sits and walks and how he moves his head and arms; also notice the expressions on his face and the sound of his voice. Now imagine you are that person – that shape and size, with that voice. What would things be like if you were that person? How would it feel if you moved that way or spoke that way?

Before we leave this section, there is a final exercise on shifts of perspective. This is to do with being able both to distance yourself from things and to immerse yourself in them.

For this exercise, sit with this book and really notice how it feels in your hand. Pay attention to its weight, the surface of the pages, how they sound as you turn them, how the white spaces between the printed lines look and how you feel, right now, as you sit in the chair and read the book.

Now, imagine that someone has come into the room with a video camera and is filming you, right now. Then imagine how you would look on the video when it is played back. How would you be sitting? What position would your head be in? How quickly would you be turning the pages? What expression would you have on your face?

Doing this exercise helps you experience things in two ways. The first part helps you become aware of the **sensations** involved in reading the book. The second part helps you become aware of **what you are doing** as you read the book, ie to distance yourself from the experience, as if you were an observer.

Doing the exercises in this section will begin to give you some insights into other people's experiences and show you how the ways they behave are very connected with the 'positions' they are in; it will also help you become more self-observant.

Some of the advice I will be giving you later in the book will involve using one or other of these processes in order to achieve results.

Seeing things in a new light

This is similar, in some ways, to shifting perspective. Sometimes the process of seeing things in a new light is referred to as reframing, or putting a different slant on situations. For example, if you are ill, you could think of it as a problem, but it could also give you more time at home to catch up with reading or to get away from a stressful work environment. Thinking of the illness in these kinds of ways is reframing, or putting a different interpretation, or meaning, onto situations, events, objects or interactions.

Seeing things in a new light can be a useful skill when

considering weight control. For example, missing out on an ice cream, bar of chocolate or extra helping of pudding could be reframed as an increase in self-control. Having lost only 1lb/500g in weight could be reframed as having got half-way towards your weekly goal.

Have a go at the following exercises, which will help you later when we apply them to your weight-control process.

You are asked out to an expensive restaurant for a meal. You know there will be lots of tempting things to eat. How could you reframe this invitation in a positive way?

You hear someone make a comment about your weight which you think is not very complimentary. How could you reframe this occurrence so that you do not react badly to it?

Projecting yourself into the future

Just as you may tend to have a fixed perspective on things, you may only see things from one point in time. For example, if you are overweight at present, you may have the sense that that is how things will be for ever. If you can recall a past time when things were different, or a future time when things will be different again, it is possible to have more hope and encouragement for your efforts.

People talk of time travel as an impossible dream but, in your mind, time travel is not only possible, it is commonplace. How often have you remembered things from your childhood, or thought ahead to a future event? This is mental time travel and, by using it in a deliberate way, you can make real shifts in your thinking. The next exercise will help you work with time shifts in some exciting ways.

For this exercise, find a place where you can put an imaginary line on the floor; the line can be any length you like, but around 10ft/3m would be a good length to start with. The line will represent the past, present and future, so decide which end will be the past and which will be the future; the present will be somewhere between, wherever you feel it should be.

Now think of a future event which you are looking forward to. Stand on the line in the place you have decided will represent the present time. From there, look along the line towards the future end. Somewhere at that end, imagine yourself at a time when the event is happening; really picture yourself in the event and see how you would look. Notice your shape and notice how you would be standing or moving; notice the expression you would have on your face.

Now walk along the line towards the image you have pictured and stand in that spot, facing the same direction your imaginary self was facing. From that position, notice what it feels like to be really experiencing that future event. Notice how your body feels, what your posture is like, what your breathing is like, what expression you have on your face. Now look around you and notice the surroundings you will be in during that future event. If there are other people there, notice how they are behaving too. Become aware of how good it feels to be in that situation, even though it is just in your mind at present.

We will be returning to this kind of exercise later in the book as doing this sort of 'time shift' can give you additional resources by creating real motivation to achieve the things you desire. Even though the event is still imaginary, once you have created it as if it were real, your mind believes it has actually happened already, and begins to draw you towards it in reality.

By the way, the idea of moving yourself into the future to experience your goals is a very old one. Writers on self-development generally put forward the principle that if you imagine yourself having achieved a goal, and really allow your mind to experience what that is like, it becomes incredibly enticing and really draws you towards it – because the thought is operating at an unconscious level and acting directly on your mind. Some exciting books which tell you more about the techniques for using your mind to help draw you towards goals are listed in the Bibliography.

Self-triggers

Finally, here is one last exercise, which will help you control your feelings effectively – a useful skill when managing your responses to eating and exercising.

This exercise is based on a naturally occurring process. You will probably have had times in your life when certain things have triggered off memories, for example, hearing a particular piece of music and being reminded of where you were and who you were with when you first heard it. We will be going through a similar process now, but this time *you* will be controlling the experience, rather than something from outside stimulating the memory.

So, find somewhere comfortable and quiet to sit down, where you will not be interrupted. Now, think

41

back to a time when you felt very motivated to do something; perhaps to go on a holiday, to finish a piece of work, to meet someone, to learn something, or anything else you care to choose.

Recreate that time in your mind. Really experience it by thinking about where you were at the time, what you could see (what objects, shapes and colours), what you could hear (the loudness of sounds or the quietness of the place), what smells, what tastes, what physical sensations (how warm or cool you were; whether you were holding or touching anything; whether you were sitting, standing, moving or lying down), whether you were saying anything to yourself in your head (and if so, how loudly and what tone of voice you were using) and how it felt being really motivated. (Did you have a feeling in your stomach, or your head, or all over? And how were you breathing – quickly or slowly, high up or low down in your rib cage?)

Once you have really recreated the feeling of motivation, press one of your big toes against the floor as you sit in your chair. (Do not stay with the feeling; just press your toe down as soon as the feeling comes to you.)

Now repeat the exercise in full. Have a stretch, then go on to the next part.

This time, press your toe against the floor and allow the feeling of motivation to come back to you as you give yourself that signal.

Doing this exercise will give you a way of choosing to feel motivated whenever you need, simply by using the toe signal. I will be discussing this process again later in the book and suggesting some more signals you can use for other resourceful states.

In this chapter, I have covered several techniques designed to help you with mental flexibility and motivation. Once you have spent a little time on the exercises, you should find you are beginning to extend your powers of managing your thoughts – a vital first step in your weight-control programme. And being able to see things in a new light should begin to show you new ways of taking steps towards your goals. If you have felt, in the past, that you could not make changes or did not know what it would be like if you succeeded, you will now have ways of recognizing that personal change is perfectly possible and that you will be able to handle things really well as you go along.

In the next chapter I will tell you much more about motivation and preferences, and will go on to give you ways of identifying, and working with, your own patterns in order to achieve results.

3
Motivation and Preferences

This chapter will explain what motivation is, how people become motivated and how motivation may be reduced or increased. It then goes on to help you work out some of your own motivation and preference patterns through some simple tests.

Understanding motivation

Motivation is the force which drives us towards goals. You will recognize motivation in your own life as a desire for achievement, as a sense of urgency about making changes or as enthusiasm for pursuing a course of action.

When you are motivated you strive to reach your desired outcomes in a purposeful and directed manner. Motivation ensures that you keep on track, maintain a sense of direction, focus your efforts on positive action and manage to overcome obstacles which might lie in your path.

It is easy to be motivated to achieve something you enjoy, but it is also possible to be motivated to take action which you do not necessarily enjoy, in order to achieve a longer-term aim. So you might endure a lengthy journey in difficult conditions if, at the end, you arrive at a pleasant and inviting location. You might pay a visit to a dentist in order to alleviate toothache or queue in the rain for several hours in order to buy some tickets for an event you particularly want to attend. Motivation is the driving force which enables us to keep going until we achieve the desired result.

The factors which motivate people are many and varied. There are many theories of motivation, which are well known in the field of business management. These theories tend to group people according to the factors which motivate them. For example one theory (Mc-Clelland) says there are three factors which motivate people: the need for power, the need for achievement and the need for social contact with other people. Another (Vroom) says that people are motivated when they have an *expectation* that their efforts will be rewarded (although the actual rewards which individuals appreciate can differ considerably).

All the motivation theories add to our store of knowledge and information but, in the end, the fact is that everyone is different and, despite the theories, motivation is an extremely personal and individual matter.

Understanding how people become motivated

The motivation theories propose that different *things* motivate people, but they tend not to have the answers regarding *how* people become motivated. In other words the theories often relate to the *content* of motivation (what it is) rather than the *process* (how it happens).

NLP, which I introduced you to in the last chapter, offers some very simple ideas about *how* people become motivated. In essence, the principle is that motivation occurs when the mind produces thoughts which direct your attention towards a goal in a particular way.

These thoughts are produced through your senses (sight, hearing, touch, taste and smell) to produce images, sounds and other 'internal representations', and I hope you have already experimented with these in the exercises in the last chapter.

I will be showing you how to use these processes in your own programme in chapter 5. The general principle is that there is a difference between what your mind does when you are motivated and what it does when you are not motivated, and these differences vary from person to person. By analysing your own mental patterns for motivation and lack of motivation, you can develop an understanding of what to do to harness your mental powers in a positive and effective manner.

Understanding what can reduce or increase motivation

In the previous chapter, we considered five elements which contribute to success: goals, thoughts, feelings, beliefs and behaviour. These same factors affect motivation.

For example, having a clear goal can be very motivating, whereas a fuzzy goal is harder to be inspired by. An objective which seems attainable can be very motivating, whereas one which seems unattainable may well demotivate you.

Positive *thinking* can be motivating; for example *picturing* things going well, or *telling yourself* positive things about what you can achieve. You may, in the past, have done the opposite of this and told yourself you were likely to fail, or pictured things going wrong.

Similarly, you can create positive feelings or negative

ones. When you have positive thoughts you are more likely to feel good; and feeling good is more likely to produce positive thoughts. So your thoughts and feelings are closely interlinked and work together to motivate or demotivate you.

Positive beliefs are also more supportive of positive thoughts and feelings, whereas negative beliefs tend to be more limiting. Rewards are important here as, for most people, having a sense of what you will gain by succeeding is highly motivational, whereas believing that success will be accompanied by unwanted consequences is more likely to put you off .

Finally, knowing you have the skills or ability to do certain things can really help you in your quest for success, whereas it is harder to be successful if you do not know what to do, or have not worked to develop the skills needed.

In the next part of this chapter, I will be taking some specific motivational and preference patterns and discussing how these affect the ways in which you become enthusiastic about things. In order to do this, there are a few simple tests for you to do to find out what your own motivational and preference patterns are. I hope you enjoy these; they are fun to do and will give you some interesting information about yourself.

Working out your own motivational and preference patterns

I have already explained that people can have different patterns underlying their behaviour. These patterns tend to be repeated in similar situations, but can vary over time, or from context to context.

Some people have remarkably stable patterns, while others can change much more frequently. The following tests are designed to give you an idea of your own patterns, especially in relation to weight loss, but since these can change you should, from time to time, review how you actually respond in different situations.

I will be taking ten different patterns and showing you how to assess where you are in relation to each of them. For each pattern, you will find a few simple questions. You should answer these as honestly as you can; nobody but you need see the answers and doing the test accurately will definitely help you with your weight control programme. Most questions have only two possible answers, A or B, and the most helpful thing is for you to choose between these two extremes by saying which is most like you. If you feel you would have to answer somewhere between A and B for any particular question, or that you would not have chosen either of those responses, then you can move on to the next question, but please do try to answer as many as you can, because this will give you a more realistic assessment of your own patterns. Where a question has more than two options, again choose only one in each case.

The tests are divided into two groups; there are five initial sets of questions, and you will then find the answers to them explained. Then there are a further five sets of questions, with the answers to them following on. The explanations will show you how knowing about your motivation and preference patterns can help you succeed in losing weight. It is important to complete each whole set of five tests before looking at the explanations.

Remember: there are no right or wrong answers, just different ones.

PATTERN ONE

1 **When you think about things you have done in your life, do you think:**
   A you have been generally highly motivated
   B your motivation has been low, or wavered

2 **When you think about losing weight do you:**
   A feel really enthusiastic, right now, about doing it
   B think you should be doing it, but not really feel very keen on making a start

3 **Do you find you prefer to:**
   A get involved in initiating lots of things
   B leave things to others for much of the time

4 **Do you generally:**
   A start things yourself
   B wait for someone else to push you into doing things

5 **Would you find it:**
   A easy to exercise
   B hard to get going

6 **Do you usually:**
   A keep going on projects once you have started
   B find your enthusiasm wanes rather quickly

7 **Do you find:**
   A you are rarely deflected from things you take on
   B you easily get diverted into other things

PATTERN TWO

1 **Do you tend to:**
   A analyse things you have done and what went well or badly
   B just get on with the next thing that comes along

2 **Do you generally:**
   A decide on a course of action because it seems the most logical thing to do
   B make a decision based on how quickly you can put it into practice

3 **Do you usually:**
   A think about doing things, but often put them off
   B get on with them straight away

4 **Do you tend to:**
   A think things through thoroughly before taking action
   B jump in without much thought

5 **Do you prefer to:**
   A understand the principles of how things work before you do anything
   B have a go first and then find out how things work

6 **Do you prefer to:**
   A read about new weight control programmes
   B try them out

7 **Do you like:**
   A planning things out in your mind
   B making a start and seeing how things go

PATTERN THREE

1 **When you think about losing weight do you:**
   A think about how you were in the past
   B notice how you are right now
   C look forward to how you will be in the future

2 **When you consider your food do you:**
   A remember what you had yesterday that you shouldn't have

B think about what you are eating today

C plan what you will eat tomorrow

3 **Which of the following best describes you?**

A I rely on past experience to guide what I do.

B I just react to how things are at the moment.

C I think about the future consequences of the things I do.

4 **When you think about your weight, do you:**

A think the future has to be like the past

B get so concerned about how you are right now that you cannot imagine anything different

C think the future is a new experience

5 **Do you prefer:**

A stories about how people have succeeded at things in the past

B stories about how people are achieving things right now

C stories about how people set their goals and direction for the future

6 **If you have a problem, do you:**

A think about how you tackled similar things in the past

B deal with it in the best way you know right now

C work out how to avoid it happening again in the future

7 **Do you think your success is affected most by:**

A how successful you have been in the past at getting results

B what you do right now to achieve results

C how well you can work towards your goals in the future

PATTERN FOUR

1 **Which describes you best?**
   A I often make mental images of things; for example picturing things going well or badly.
   B I often imagine the things people say about me, or recall conversations I have had with people.
   C I often find myself feeling strong emotions.
   D I often 'talk to myself' in my head.

2 **Which of the following would you rather do?**
   A watch an exercise videowatch an exercise video
   B listen to an exercise audiotape or CD
   C play a sport, dance or go to a gym
   D talk yourself through a relaxation technique

3 **Which of the following would indicate to you that your weight is right?**
   A You look the way you want.
   B People tell you you look good.
   C You feel good about your weight.
   D You know in your own mind your weight is right.

4 **Do you learn most easily when:**
   A someone demonstrates what to do
   B someone tells you what to do
   C you are helped to try something out for yourself
   D you can think out what needs to be done

5 **Do you prefer cookery books which:**
   A have lots of pictures of the finished meals
   B tell you the full instructions
   C give you a feel for how the recipe will turn out
   D give you lots of ideas to think about

6 **If you bought some walking shoes from a catalogue, would you prefer:**
   A to see a picture of the shoes
   B to have a written description of them
   C to know how they would feel on you
   D to consider the pros and cons of the features they had

7 **Would you be most likely to assess your confidence levels by:**
   A looking in the mirror
   B hearing what other people say about you
   C noticing how you feel
   D telling yourself that you are confident

PATTERN FIVE

1 **When you hear of a new approach to weight control do you:**
   A wonder if it is as good as it sounds
   B rush to try it

2 **Do you:**
   A keep to the same basic range of foods and ways of cooking
   B like to try out new products and recipes

3 **With exercise, would you:**
   A wait until a new exercise programme, eg steps, has become generally accepted before trying it
   B have a go at anything new which comes along

4 **If you haven't succeeded with something in the past, do you think:**
   A I'd better not do that again
   B There must be something I can try to get it right.

5 **If you were given a new programme to follow, would you think:**
   A I should be really careful about making any changes in it.
   B I can do it my own way and vary what I have been told.

6 **If a friend told you of a different way of cooking food, would you think:**
   A I'm not sure it will be any good.
   B I must try that.

7 **When you buy clothes, do you:**
   A usually stick to things you know suit you
   B often try out different colours and styles

Checking your results

When you have completed the first five tests, just add up the number of As, Bs, Cs and Ds in each pattern. The letter with the highest score in any of the tests indicates which is most typical of you and you should then read the guidance below for that response. If you find you have two scores the same in any section, your answers are evenly balanced and you should read the guidance for both, as each could apply to you at different times. It is this knowledge of your own individual patterns which will help you to control your weight.

It is important to stress again that there are no 'good' or 'bad' answers here. It is not better or worse to fall into one category or another, although it may be that different categories are more or less useful in particular situations. So, in assessing your own scores, do remember that they are simply rough guides to your preferred ways of doing things and that you can use this information to be more effective in what you do.

So here are the explanations of the first five sets of questions, which will explain what your answers indicate about you.

PATTERN ONE: MOTIVATIONAL LEVEL

This pattern explains whether you are generally highly motivated or not, especially in relation to losing weight.

If you scored more As than Bs in this section you tend to be highly motivated and more likely to be self-motivated; if you scored more Bs than As you tend to be less well motivated and may need help from others in motivating yourself.

If you rated yourself as highly motivated you will probably continue to have high motivation to follow the approach set out in this book. If you rated yourself as having low motivation you may need some extra assistance in getting started on a new programme. Many of the exercises in the book are specially designed to increase and enhance motivation and you should find them really useful in making changes in your life.

PATTERN TWO: PREFERENCE FOR THINKING OR TAKING ACTION

This pattern explains whether you tend to spend a good deal of time thinking, or prefer to get into action quickly.

If you scored more As than Bs in this section your pattern is 'thinking'; if you scored more Bs than As it is 'doing'.

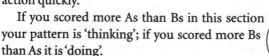

'Thinking' people spend a good deal of time 'in

their head'. If this is like you, you will probably like to work things out and to plan. You may spend quite a bit of time considering the implications of things before taking action. The result can sometimes be that your ideas may not always get turned into reality.

'Doing' people like getting on with things. If this is like you, you will probably prefer to jump in and have a go rather than spend time analysing options. You may, however, give up on things because you have not thought them out in advance or, when you get into them, you may find that they are not quite as you had anticipated.

PATTERN THREE: TIME

This pattern explains whether you tend to 'live in' the past, present or future.

If you scored mostly As in this section you are often likely to hark back to the past; if you scored mostly Bs you tend to live more in the present and if you scored mostly Cs you tend to be more future focused.

People who incline to the past may have either positive or negative thoughts about events which have occurred. If the thoughts are negative, they may remember how they used to be and can find it hard to believe that they are now different, or they may remember not succeeding in making changes in the past and find it difficult to think that they can make them in the future.

Those who live in the present are very conscious of how things are right now. If this is like you, you may be good at assessing what needs to be done, but may find it difficult to think of a time when change will have happened.

Future-orientated people look ahead and often think about how things will be, or how they would like them to be. If this is like you, you may sometimes look ahead and anticipate things going well, but at other times you may see problems coming towards you. A difficulty with future orientation is that, although you may have a good sense of where you want to be, you might put things off.

PATTERN FOUR: USING DIFFERENT SENSES

This pattern explains whether you have a preference for using one particular sense.

Each of these categories involves different senses. It is generally held that we have five senses: sight, hearing, touch, taste and smell (and a sub-category of hearing is when we talk to ourselves in our heads, hearing imaginary sounds). The categories here deal with the senses of seeing, hearing (including self-talk) and feeling, as these are the senses you are likely to use most.

If you scored mostly As in this section you probably need visual stimulation if things are to keep your attention. If you scored mostly Bs you are probably influenced by what you hear, and possibly by what you read; talking things through with people may also be helpful to you. If you scored mostly Cs you are probably strongly influenced by your feelings and may respond well to things which make you feel good (this may include tactile things as well as emotional ones). If you scored mostly Ds, you probably need to think things through in your mind; possibly telling yourself about their pros and cons.

PATTERN FIVE: ATTITUDE TOWARDS NEW THINGS

This pattern explains whether you are likely to be cautious or experimental. If you scored more As than Bs in this section your pattern is 'cautious'; if you scored more Bs than As your pattern is 'experimental'.

Cautious people like to be well armed with the facts and solid evidence before they act. If this is like you, you may need to be convinced about things. You might dislike change unless it can be proved to be necessary. A difficulty with being cautious is that you may fail to make a needed change because you are afraid of the consequences of it going wrong or not living up to expectations.

Experimental people like to try things out. If this is like you, you may get bored with routine and convention and prefer to venture onto new ground. A possible problem with being experimental is that you may not stay with a process for long enough for it to work well and you may be tempted to play around with, and alter, things in ways which are not beneficial.

You have now had the first five patterns explained and I hope you will have learned some useful things about yourself and your reactions to situations. You can now move on to the second set of questions, which have the same format as the first set; ie you should select the answers which are most like you and, where possible, answer all the questions.

PATTERN SIX

1 How do you know when you look good?
   A Other people tell you.
   B You just know, inside yourself.

2 How do you know you have chosen a good outfit?
   A People compliment you on it.
   B You like it yourself.

3 How do you know what your weight should be?

A The charts say that is the correct weight for your height.

B You feel it is right for you.

4 **If someone criticizes you, do you feel:**
   A They must be right.
   B They don't know what they are talking about.

5 **If you have a particular opinion:**
   A are you easily persuaded to change it
   B do you defend it at all costs

6 **Do you want to lose weight because:**
   A other people say you should
   B you yourself believe you should

7 **How would you be most likely to decide when to exercise?**
   A Your family or friends push you into it.
   B You feel like doing it.

PATTERN SEVEN

1 **Would you prefer to:**
   A exercise on your own
   B join in a class with others

2 **Do you enjoy:**
   A eating alone
   B having a meal with friends

3 **Would you find it more helpful to:**
   A follow your own weight-control programme by yourself
   B share weight-losing experiences with a friend and help each other along

4 **Do you prefer to shop for clothes:**
   A on your own
   B with a friend

5 **Would you prefer to:**
   A assess how you are doing in your weight-control programme by yourself
   B discuss your progress with a friend

6 **If you went to a swimming pool or gym and nobody else was there, would you be more likely to:**
   A make a start on your own
   B wait until the other people arrived

7 **Are you more likely to:**
   A work through this book by yourself
   B persuade a friend to go through the activities with you

PATTERN EIGHT

1 **If you joined a fitness class, would it be more important to you that:**
   A it had useful facilities
   B it was not in an unpleasant environment

2 **If someone asks you to do something, are you more likely to respond positively if:**
   A they offer you a reward
   B they tell you they will be upset if you do not do it

3 **If you went to a weight-control class, would it be more important to you that you:**
   A got on well with the other people there
   B avoided a place where people might criticize you in some way

4 **If you cooked a meal for friends, would it be more important to you that:**
   A they complimented you on your cooking
   B nobody left any food on the plate

5 **If you bought an exercise bicycle, would it be more important to you that:**
   A it had lots of new features
   B it was not complicated to use

6 **If you have things to do, do you:**
   A do them quickly so that they can be finished
   B keep putting them off until you cannot avoid them any longer

7 **What is most important to you:**
   A looking energetic
   B not looking tired

PATTERN NINE

1 **On your desk, dressing table or bathroom shelf:**
   A does everything have its right place
   B do you just put things anywhere

2 **When you use a recipe do you:**
   A try to follow it exactly
   B improvise in your own way

3 **When you take up a new activity do you:**
   A want to be told how it should be done
   B want to be able to choose how to do it

4 **If a friend had a clothes label sticking out of the back of her collar, would you:**
   A notice it quickly and adjust it
   B not notice it, or not be concerned about it showing

5 Do you like things to be:
   A orderly and predictable
   B flexible and spontaneous

6 When buying new clothes do you tend to:
   A buy the first item which seems right for the purpose
   B seek out lots of choices to select from

7 If you read a weight-control book do you:
   A read it from start to finish as the author intended
   B skip to the bits that interest you most

PATTERN TEN

1 If you were told of a new shop which sells good food products would you:
   A need to know exactly how to get there, street names, landmarks and so forth
   B just need a rough idea of where it is

2 If you asked a friend what he had been doing that day, would you:
   A want to know everything that had happened
   B prefer a short summary

3 If you asked someone to get you a food product from a supermarket, would you:
   A tell him exactly what brand, size, price, etc
   B give him an idea of what you want and then leave it to him to select

4 If you had to assemble a new piece of exercise equipment would you:
   A need detailed instructions
   B only need to know the general principles of what goes where

5 **If you asked someone in your family to help support you during your programme, would you:**
   A tell him precisely what to do
   B just give him an outline of what you want

6 **If you went to an exercise class, would you:**
   A have to have each movement explained precisely
   B just need to know the overall purpose of the exercise

7 **When you hear that a particular food is supposed to be healthy, do you:**
   A need to know exactly why
   B just accept the fact with a minimum of evidence

Checking your results

The following pages give you explanations of the second five patterns. As I said earlier, there are no 'good' or 'bad' patterns, but there are situations where one or another pattern can be more appropriate.

For example, pattern six deals with the degree to which you are independent in your thoughts and behaviour, in other words whether you find it easy to make your own decisions and judgements. If you are in a car and get a puncture, it is probably more useful to be able to make your own decision to pull over to one side than to have to ask someone else what to do; safety here is likely to depend on rapid responses. If, however, your family is taking a holiday, it might be better to pay attention to what the others want to do, rather than just make the decisions yourself without any consultation. So bear in mind, as you read the explanations, that your own patterns will be very useful at times, but could be counter-productive at others.

PATTERN SIX: SELF-RELIANCE

This pattern explains whether you rely heavily on your own opinions or prefer to have feedback and support from others. If you scored more As than Bs, your pattern is 'external' (less self-reliant). If you scored more Bs than As your pattern is 'internal' (more self-reliant).

'External' people tend to need feedback and support from others. If this is like you, you may sometimes be easily swayed by other people's opinions and influenced to believe that your own opinions are incorrect. Because of a need for others' acknowledgement, you may lack confidence and self-esteem and be reluctant to do anything unless someone else says it is all right to do it.

'Internal' people are often independent and rely heavily on their own ideas and opinions. If this is like you, you will probably tend to have strongly held opinions which you defend energetically. You are likely to be self-motivated and self-determining. You probably do not easily listen to, or accept, other people's views unless you can somehow evaluate them and decide they fit in with how you think or what you believe. You may be so self-opinionated that you do not take any advice and may miss out on things which could help you.

PATTERN SEVEN: SOCIABILITY

This pattern explains whether you prefer to do things on your own or with other people. It is similar to pattern six, but is more about whether you *like* being with others, rather than whether you *need* others to help you make decisions.

If you scored more As than Bs in this section you are

'intrapersonal' (doing things on your own); if you scored more Bs than As you are 'interpersonal' (doing things with others).

'Intrapersonal' people like doing things on their own. If this is like you, you can do very well when left to your own devices and you may find being with others is stressful or you may simply find you get more done if you can be by yourself. Doing things on your own can be very productive, but it may mean you only get a one-sided view of things. It may also mean you lack support from others at times when it could be very helpful.

'Interpersonal' people like doing things with other people. If this is like you, you may get lonely if left to your own devices and you probably like the interaction involved in being with other people. Needing to be with others can mean you are never short of company, but it can also mean you rarely get time to yourself to explore what you really need.

PATTERN EIGHT: DIRECTION OF MOTIVATION

This pattern explains whether you are goal-seeking or problem-avoiding. If you scored more As than Bs in this section, your pattern is goal-seeking (sometimes called a 'towards' pattern); if you scored more Bs than As your pattern is problem-avoiding (sometimes called an 'away from' pattern).

Goal-seeking people are motivated by achieving goals. If this is like you, you will enjoy getting results and working towards the things you want. You may sometimes not see obstacles because you are so focused on your goals. This is good in one way, because it means you are likely to be very persistent and single-minded in working towards what you want, but it can also mean you may run into trouble because you have not anticipated possible problems.

Problem-avoiding people are motivated by avoiding or overcoming problems and getting away from difficulties. If this is like you, you may tend to see the pitfalls in situations and be good at trouble-shooting. You may, however, be so conscious of difficulties to overcome that you sometimes find it hard to work towards a goal.

PATTERN NINE: DEGREE OF FLEXIBILITY

This pattern explains whether you prefer to follow set paths or have lots of choices. If you scored more As than Bs in this section, your pattern is 'rules'; if you scored more Bs than As your pattern is 'options'.

'Rules' people like to have set ways of doing things. If this is like you, you are likely to be orderly and systematic. You may get upset if things are changed around or altered. You probably like to know where you stand and what is expected of you. A possible problem for you is that you may not be able to step outside a system if things do not go as expected and you may find it difficult to know what action to take if you do not have a set route to follow.

'Options' people like flexibility and choice. If this is like you, you will probably like to be able to do things in whatever way seems appropriate at the time, without being constrained by previous con-ventions. You will not mind if there is no system in place, or if it breaks down, as you can still function effectively 'playing things by ear'. You may, however, be so keen on trying out new things that you do not settle on anything in particular and find it hard to stay on track.

PATTERN TEN: LEVEL OF DETAIL NEEDED

This pattern explains whether you need lots of detail or prefer to have an overview, or more general outline, of things you are involved in. If you scored more As than Bs in this section your pattern is that of 'detail'; if you scored more Bs than As your pattern is 'general'.

'Detail' people, as the term suggests, like detail. If this is like you, you will probably need a lot of information about things before you can function well. You like to work things out so you know how they fit together. You may find it hard to perform well unless you have enough information before you start something. Sometimes, you may spend so much time collecting detailed information that you do not see the general principles involved and fail to understand the general direction in which you should be going.

'General' people can get frustrated with detail. If this is like you, you probably work well when you have a general idea of what to do and how to set about it. You are likely to take an overview of things and may often talk in generalizations. You are likely to work very well with principles as guidance rather than needing to have specific instructions. A possible difficulty is that you may fail to get the detail right, and not quite achieve the goal you set out to, because you leave small, but important, elements undone.

The important thing to remember with all these categories is that they are only *underlying* patterns, they do not necessarily determine the results you actually get in life. So, for example, a problem-avoiding person (pattern eight) may actually be very good at working to achieve a goal, but will do so *to get away from a problem* rather than to achieve the goal itself.

Now you have spent some time exploring your own motivational patterns; in the next chapter I will show you how to use this knowledge in your own personal weight-control programme. I will be taking a look at what you can do, in a practical way, to make changes, taking into account the unique patterns which make up your own personality.

4
Making It Real

> Now you have discovered some of your
> motivational and preference patterns, you can
> move on to finding out how to use this
> information in making your weight-control
> programme really successful. When you use
> methods which fit with your own ways of
> achieving things, it is much easier to get results
> and also enjoy what you are doing.

What 'making it real' means

The title of this chapter has two meanings. The first is
that, by taking action, you bring your plans to reality and
give life to them. But there is a second meaning, which is
also important.

For many people, weight control is an *idea*. It is something they have in the back of their minds, or something
they talk to their friends about. It is something they read
about in magazines. It is something they wish they had
done. It is something they hope to do in the future. But,
somehow, it is not 'real'. What I mean by this is that they
do not have anything in their minds which gives them
the feeling of what it would be like to succeed.

Let me explain this further. Suppose there is something you really, really want to do – for example, going
on a particular holiday. As you think about the holiday
you might be seeing in your mind the place you intend
to visit; maybe picturing the colour of the sky, trees

waving in the breeze, and sun shining on white roofs. Perhaps you imagine the sound of waves coming in and breaking on a sandy shore, or the sound of seagulls shrieking as they fly overhead. Possibly you imagine the scent of wild flowers or the taste of tropical fruit. You might also imagine the feel of sand between your toes and the excitement of being in a wonderful location with time to do all the things you want.

When you use your mind in this way you are actually creating, not just a mental image, but a *real sensation* of something which will happen in the future. Your mind actually believes this event will occur; it is like imagining the taste of a lemon in your mouth; although the lemon is not really there, your mind thinks it is and makes your mouth water.

And when you give your mind this kind of experience it is very enticing and draws you towards it. So if you are serious about losing weight, you will need to get your mind to help you. By allowing your mind to create sensations of the future *as if they are real*, you will find yourself becoming motivated to achieve them. And this is *very different* from just having the idea that you will lose weight, or just talking to your friends about what you want to achieve.

This chapter and the following one are designed to show you how to use your mind in this way, actively harnessing its power in support of your goals. Everyone can use their minds positively; you just need to know how. It may be that in the past you have used your mind in a negative way – allowing it to produce sensations of things going badly – but, once you know how, you can reverse this and have your mind work *for* you in an enjoyable and effective way.

The next chapter will give you ways of making positive changes, especially in how you think. In particular, it will help you think more positively, by making positive images in your mind, by hearing positive sounds and by having positive feelings. What you will be practising are some of the techniques I introduced you to in chapter 2, and you will learn ways of making real changes in how you think, so you can achieve the results you want. But, before we move on to the actual changes you can make, this chapter will concentrate on helping you identify what you are doing at present in relation to your weight, and what you would like to be doing instead. This advice applies to everyone, so you should read it through before moving on to chapter 5.

You will probably find it useful to have a pen and paper with you for both this chapter and the next one, as some of the things you will be doing involve making notes of situations or listing things which are important to you. Take as long as you need to work through the exercises, there is no need to hurry, just take things at your own pace. And if you think it would be more useful to work through them with a friend, then just get someone else to help you; or, better still, do the exercises together (although your friend will also have to complete the tests in chapter 3 before doing these exercises with you).

Where you are now and where you would like to be

What we are moving on to now is comparing how things are for you now (your **present state**) with how you would like them to be in the future (your **desired state**).

I talked in chapter 2 about the different things which

have an impact on the results you get. Just to remind you, they are: your goals, your behaviour, the way you think, the way you feel and the beliefs you have. I will now take each of these elements in turn, so you can work out what you are doing at present and what you could do instead with regard to each of them. Then, as I have already mentioned, you will be going on in the next chapter to find out exactly how you can achieve the results you are aiming for.

Take some time to sit quietly and read through the following sections. As you read each one, think carefully about your own present situation. See how many of the things mentioned apply to you. If the specific examples are not relevant, simply substitute ones which would be more useful. Then go on to consider what you would prefer to have in each of the areas.

You may choose to do this in your head but, as I have already recommended, it might be best for you to write down your thoughts about each section on sheets of paper. This will be helpful in thinking it through and will also be useful later on when you come to make changes. When you have achieved your results, you can look back and compare what you have achieved with how things were before, and really notice the difference.

GOALS

Present state

You may have some very sensible and appropriate goals which you want to work towards, but you could also have some goals which are not so good. Some people aim for things which are impossible; are you among them? See if any of these apply to you.

- I want to look exactly as I did ten years go.
- I want to look like a supermodel.
- I want to continue eating everything I want and also lose weight.
- I want a 'quick-fix' plan which will change my weight in a matter of days.
- I want to lose weight without exercising.
- I want to lose weight by exercise alone, without having to change my eating habits.

Think about any other unrealistic goals you have and list these as well.

Now, before we move on to considering some more useful goals you might set, let's just spend a few minutes considering how you might approach goal setting in general.

Goal setting

First of all, it helps to have very specific goals. So you might have a goal of going to an exercise class once a week, or of losing 2lb/1kg of weight a week, or walking up all the stairs in your office instead of taking the lift, or eating some fresh vegetables each day.

Here are some simple pointers which can help you make sure your goals are well thought out.

- **Make them positive.** This means saying what you do want, rather than what you do not. So, it is better to say, 'I want to eat some fresh vegetables each day', rather than 'I don't want to eat crisps or snacks.' Putting your goals into positive language will help you reach your targets. When you say what you do not want, it is hard to know what to aim for; far better to be precise about what your actual target is.

- **Make them specific and measurable.** This means setting them out in detail and having ways of assessing how far you have gone towards achieving your results. So you might say, 'I want to lose 2lb/1kg a week', or 'I want to spend 20 minutes exercising three times a week' or 'I want to be able to run for 15 minutes without getting out of breath.' The more detail you use in specifying the goals and standards you want to aim for, the easier it is to check your progress.
- **Make them realistic and achievable.** This means having goals which are within your reach: not too difficult and not too easy. It is all right having easy goals to start with, but you will benefit more if you make them progressively more challenging as you work through your programme, although they should not be set so high that you become demotivated in trying to achieve them. So be realistic and set your-self goals which are somewhat challenging, but still achievable. If you are not sure what is an appropriate level to set, do get help from someone who is well informed about diet and exercise; this may be a fitness coach, nutritionist, your doctor or another similar professional.
- **Have a time scale for them.** This means setting yourself some measure to do with time. There are a range of measures which you could choose; some of these are:

  - when you will start the activity
  - when you will complete the activity
  - how long you will spend on the activity
  - how often you will do the activity

Probably a good way of approaching this to start with is to give yourself a frequency and a duration; for example: 'I will go to my exercise class twice a week for the next three months.' So the frequency is twice a week and the completion time is three months. You can choose to alter the frequency, to extend the completion time or to alter the activity itself at any time, but at least you have a starting point from which to assess your progress.

- **Make sure they fit with who you are.** This means that it really helps to set goals that fit with your self-image and your lifestyle. It is no use having goals that are fine for other people but are not right for you; you probably will not retain the motivation to work for them. For example, suppose you are keen to go to an exercise class to keep fit, but the class you select is on a Wednesday evening and your job as a sales representative means you have to travel most weeks to see customers. Although you may really want to go to the class, your lifestyle at present makes it difficult to fit in. So, although the goal in itself is a good one, it does not fit with the way you live at present, and you would be better off choosing another goal which could achieve similar results while still fitting in with the rest of your life.

- **Make sure you have the resources to achieve them.** This means checking that this is the right time to do what you have in mind. For example, do you have the time to spend on exercise programmes, do you have the money to spend on fitness classes, do you have the support from friends to keep you motivated, do you have the information you need to get started? Some of these may not be necessary; for example you could walk more, which does not cost anything, or you could motivate yourself rather than needing anyone else to help you with it. But working these things out in advance is useful as it allows you to check what you need before you start, and then to plan to make it possible.

- **Make sure you work out the pros and cons of achieving them.** This is the one which is most likely to keep you on track. Often, people set goals which they think they want but, if they are really honest, would involve either giving up things they really value or making changes which would have undesirable consequences. For example, to lose weight you may have to eat less of certain foods which you really like or you may have to turn down things your friends are having. You may also find that, if your weight were different, people would have different perceptions and expectations of you which you might not like, such as expecting you always to dress smartly or to make speeches at events because you look so confident. So, working out the consequences of either staying the same or changing is important; once you know what is involved you can give it your full commitment or decide it is not for you.

Desired state

Having considered goal setting in general, what are some specific goals which you might want to substitute for the ones you had previously? Think about the following and see if any of them would be suitable goals for you.

- I would like to be of average weight, for a person of my height, in six months' time.
- I would like to be a similar weight to what I was a year ago by the time my summer holiday comes.

- I would like to be able to get into clothes one size smaller by the end of October.
- I would like to eat three vegetables a day, every day.
- I would like to walk to work, instead of driving, three times a week.

Do any of these sound good to you? And are there other goals you would like to achieve? If so, just add them, or substitute them for some of the goals listed above.

This section will have helped you understand how to set goals and how to change inappropriate goals into more useful ones. You can now move on to the next part, which is about encouraging your mind to work well for you.

THOUGHTS

Present state

Take a few moments to think about how things are for you right now, in relation to your weight. As you do this, *pay attention* to the thoughts going through your mind. As I said earlier, some of the things which go to make up thoughts are mental images and imaginary sounds, tastes and smells. Notice which of these come into your mind as you think about your present weight, your present eating habits, your present levels of activity and any other aspects of your life which relate, in any way, to your weight.

Now, as you pay attention to the thoughts in your mind, notice if you are doing any of the following.

- picturing yourself (possibly seeing yourself as overweight or as unfit, or seeing yourself with others and comparing yourself with them, or seeing yourself

77

eating particular foods, or seeing yourself being stared at)

- picturing other people (possibly people who you think look better than you)
- hearing other people say things (perhaps commenting on your weight or appearance, or saying they do not think you will be successful in losing weight)
- saying things to yourself (maybe telling yourself you weigh too much, or that you will never lose the weight, or that you have tried in the past and not succeeded)
- imagining tastes (maybe of particular foods you really like)
- imagining smells (perhaps of particular foods you really enjoy)

Did any other thoughts go through your mind as you did this exercise? If so, list them as well.

You have now probably found that your mind was producing images, sounds and sensations which were not all desirable.

Desired state

Now take a few minutes to consider what alternative thoughts you can create. Yes, it is perfectly possible to create thoughts just by choosing to do so – this is the main principle I am suggesting to you in this book. So what would you *like* to think about your weight? Would any of the following be helpful?

- I would like to picture myself looking good.
- I would like to imagine people complimenting me on my appearance.
- I would like to tell myself I am achieving results.

Are there any more thoughts you would *like* to have about your weight? List as many as you can here; we will be making use of them in the next chapter.

Before you move on, let us take this thought process to a more detailed level. In the following chapter, I will be giving you guidance relating to your own specific motivational patterns. But to avoid repetition, I would like to show you here just how to change the *detail* of your thoughts from things you do not want to do to things you do want to do.

Let's take the example of a food which you would prefer to avoid. When you think about that food you can imagine its taste, its smell, its texture in your mouth, its appearance, any sound it makes (such as being crunchy) and anything you might tell yourself about it. To change your mental response to it, all you need to do is to substitute different sensations in your mind. So instead of imagining the taste of that food you could imagine an alternative taste; either an appealing taste of a healthier food, which would encourage you to eat that instead, or an unpleasant taste of a different kind, which could put you off eating at all at this time.

Similarly, you could imagine a different smell, a different texture, a different appearance and a different sound. You could also imagine saying something different to yourself about the food; perhaps 'I will feel uncomfortable if I eat this' rather than 'I must eat this right now.' In the next chapter I will be showing you how to make these changes in your imagination in order to achieve the results you want.

Making these detailed changes in your mind helps you to do things differently. Please bear this process in mind as you go through this chapter and the next one;

take each of the things you find difficult at present and, in your mind, substitute something different. You will be amazed at the results this can bring.

FEELINGS

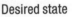

Present state

People's feelings about their weight vary. Take a little time to consider your own. Some people react to being overweight by having negative emotions, which keep them in unresourceful states; is this the case with you? For example, do any of the following feelings apply to you?

- I feel frustrated about my weight.
- I feel upset about my weight.
- I feel angry about my weight.
- I feel depressed about my weight.
- I feel helpless about my weight.
- I feel annoyed about my weight.
- I feel resigned about my weight.

Are there other feelings you have about your weight? If so, write these down too.

Desired state

Now you can move on to feelings which might be more supportive of your programme to lose weight.

What kind of feelings would you like to have about your weight? How about any of the following?

- I would like to feel good about my weight.
- I would like to have the sensation of clothes fitting me well.

- I would like to be able to feel cool and comfortable instead of hot and sticky.
- I would like to feel at ease when running for a bus, rather than getting out of breath.
- I would like to enjoy a swim and feel I look good in a swimming costume.

Are there any more feelings you would like to have about your weight? If so, add them to the list or substitute them for some of those I have mentioned.

By considering what feelings would be useful, you have made a start in your process of change. The next chapter will give you some specific ways of changing your feelings.

BEHAVIOUR

Although thoughts and feelings are important, because they give you the motivation to make changes, it is your *behaviour* which has produced your excess weight and so it is your behaviour which must change if you are to weigh less. So, let us start by considering your present behaviour.

Present state

Take a while to think very carefully about what you *do* which results in you being overweight. Different people do different things which result in them gaining weight; see if any of the following apply to you.

- I snack frequently.
- I go on food binges.
- I often eat leftovers from dishes when I have really eaten enough already.

- I eat too many sweet things.
- I drink too much alcohol.
- I eat too many fatty things.
- I eat while doing other things.
- If I have one chocolate, biscuit, etc, I always end up eating them all.

Again, add to this list if there are other things you do which increase your weight.

Keeping a food diary

Once you are clear about your behaviour, you will find it easier to make changes. An aid to this is keeping a food diary, so while you are thinking about behaviour, this could be a good time to start your diary. It is very simple; all you need to do is to take a notebook and, every day for at least a week (two weeks is better), write down in it everything you eat or drink, together with the time you ate it, where you were, what was going on, how you felt, and whether you had planned to eat then. An example of a page from such a diary is illustrated below.

You will find that a number of things happen when you keep a food diary. It will probably concentrate your

TIME	FOOD	PLACE	EVENTS	FEELINGS	PLANNED
7.45am	Orange juice Scrambled eggs Toast & butter	Home	Family getting ready to go out	Quite good	Yes
10.30am	Coffee with milk	Work	Waiting for boss to return from meeting	A little tired	Yes
11.00am	Chocolate bar	Work	Just spoken to a critical customer on the phone	Upset	No

mind, so that you become more *aware* of eating. You will also begin to notice patterns in your eating, such as the times and places you eat. You may notice associations between eating and your feelings, or connections between food and activities. And you may notice other things as well.

Two weeks is a good length of time to keep a food diary, as long as it is a fairly typical couple of weeks. Avoid picking something out of the ordinary, for example weeks with very hot weather when you do not feel like eating much anyway, or weeks with a very stressful event in them, when you may be eating more than usual just to get through the days. If you wish, keep the diary for more than two weeks to check your eating habits and to notice any changes in them.

Desired state

Now you have some ideas about monitoring your behaviour and, through this, keeping track of your thoughts and feelings, let us consider what behaviour would be more useful to you in order to achieve and maintain your correct weight.

Which of the following could be appropriate for you?

- I would like to eat more vegetables.
- I would like to exercise three times a week.
- I would like to resist the sweet puddings in restaurants and choose healthier options instead.
- I would like to keep my fridge full of healthy foods.

Are there other things you would like to do from now on? If so, make a note of them now.

This section has given you ways of assessing your present behaviour and thinking about how you might change it to more useful behaviour. Again, we will be returning to practical guidance on behaviour in the next chapter.

BELIEFS

Finally, your beliefs. We have thought about setting goals, thinking positively, feeling good and behaving in a sensible way. So, how do your beliefs affect your weight?

Present state

Take some time to think about what you believe about your present weight. Do you believe any of the following?

- I am always going to be overweight.
- I'm not the kind of person who can be successful.
- I have failed in the past, so I'm likely to do so again.
- Controlling weight is very hard work.
- I do not deserve to look good.
- My friends will not want to be with me if I do not join in what they do.
- It is impossible to manage my weight when I have to cook big meals for the family.
- I do not have time to exercise.
- I wasn't good at exercise at school, so I probably cannot do it well now.

Are there any more beliefs to add to this list? If so, add them now.

What you believe is really important, because it influences everything you do. If you have a negative belief it can make you think, feel and act negatively. It is also interesting to note that negative beliefs tend to be self-reinforcing. In other words, what you see, hear and feel tends to bear out what you believe because you are

84

'filtering out' anything which does not fit with your expectations.

Let me give you an example of this. Suppose you believe people stare at you because of your weight. You will probably notice people looking in your direction. But some of those people may simply be looking past you at something else. It is only your imagination that makes you feel they are looking at you but, if you *believe* that is what they are doing, that is what you notice.

So to change your beliefs, it helps to look for evidence that contradicts them, or to seek experiences which allow you to acquire new and useful beliefs. We shall be returning to this topic in the next chapter. In the meantime, let us see what alternative beliefs you might choose to hold.

Desired state

Would you like to believe any of the following?

- I am capable of controlling my weight.
- I will reach my target weight within six months.
- I deserve to look good.
- I can resist overeating.
- I can look good as myself without having to copy anyone else.

Are there any other things you would like to believe about yourself? Again, add as many as you would like.

This chapter will have helped you to be clearer about what you want, and about how that differs from what you have at present. You will have seen that there are many positive changes you could make and, in the next chapter, I will give you ways of making these changes. It is now time to move on and find out exactly *how* to change your patterns.

5
Steps to Take

In chapter 2, I mentioned a three-stage process; checking where you are now (present state), thinking about where you want to be (desired state) and thinking about how to get there (steps to take). Now you have thought about your present and desired states, you can move on to making changes. In this chapter, I will be showing you how *to take the steps towards achieving your goals.*

Each of the following sections is about one of the motivational and preference patterns we have been discussing. Go to whichever of the patterns your test results from chapter 3 indicate are most like you. When you get to each section, you will find a number of activities which have been designed to help you make changes in what you are doing at present. Have a go at the activities I suggest. If you need more practice at any of the techniques, turn back to chapter 2 and go through some of the exercises there again. (The pictures next to the paragraphs will correspond with the pictures in chapter 2, so you know which sections to turn to).

Remember that as well as the things I have suggested to you here, you should also add others of your own. What I have given you are simply *some* ways in which you can do things differently. So if, for example, I have shown you how to choose different items of food in a supermarket, you can add your own process for working out how to choose different items on a menu for a family meal. It is up to you to add whatever you feel would be helpful, because you are the only expert on yourself.

And if you are not convinced that the test results have revealed the 'real you', just read the other sections as well and, if you feel any of them sound more like you, then follow those instructions instead. The important thing is to have a process which works for you – and you will be the best judge of that.

Here is a general point to think about before you continue. In all the sections that follow, the exercises are designed to help you get results by using the preferences you already have. In other words the guidance relates to what you are like at present, so by following the guidance you will be helped to carry on in the ways you have already become accustomed to. In life, however, we often get more from developing than from staying the same. There is a saying which goes: 'If you always do what you've always done, you always get what you've always got.' And this is very true. So if you would like to expand your horizons and allow yourself the possibility of becoming more capable than you have been in the past, you might like to try out some new ways of doing things.

For this reason I suggest that, in each of the areas which follow, once you have worked on the guidance given, you experiment with some of the guidance given for the categories which are the opposite of your own. For example, if you are someone who enjoys doing things on your own, the exercises below will give you suggestions about how you can use this knowledge to devise activities which you can do by yourself. If, however, you also try to incorporate some activities which you can do with others instead of just by yourself, you may well find that you get benefits which had not occurred to you before, such as mutual support, feedback, new ideas and so on. So by experimenting with options, you are likely to extend your capabilities, and you may well find that this gives you fresh insights into how you can lead the rest of your life.

So my suggestion is for you to decide which is right for you, and this self-control and self-management will give you a good start in the programme because, however much you may like to have help from others, it still has to be you who eats healthily and exercises well; nobody else can do that for you.

Let me just remind you of the motivation patterns which we will be covering in this chapter. They are:

- **Motivational level.** This is about whether you find it easy or hard to get going.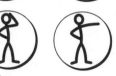
- **Preference for thinking or taking action.** This is about whether you prefer sitting and thinking or going out and taking action.
- **Time.** This is about whether you tend to live more in the past, present or future.
- **Using different senses.** This is about whether you make greater use of your senses of sight, hearing, feeling or 'internal analysis'.

- **Attitudes towards new things.** This is about whether you tend to be cautious or experimental.

- **Self-reliance.** This is about whether you need feed-back and support from others or rely on your own opinions.

- **Sociability.** This is about whether you prefer to do things on your own or with other people.

- **Direction of motivation.** This is to do with whether you prefer striving to achieve targets or avoiding problems.

- **Degree of flexibility.** This is about whether you prefer to follow set paths or have lots of options.

- **Level of detail needed.** This is about the extent to which you need informa-tion in your life.

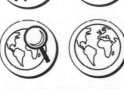

We will be taking each of these in turn, so all you need to do is turn to the relevant pages for advice. Because of the way in which the tests were designed, there will be at least one element of each pattern which applies to you, and you may find that you have elements of more than one category in some patterns. So if, for example, there are times when you like to do things on your own and times when you like to do things with other people, you can read through the advice for each and then select whichever you feel is most appropriate to follow in a particular situation.

As with chapter 3, I have divided the patterns into two groups. The first covers the first five patterns, which are rather broader in their applications. The second covers the next five, and goes into much more detail.

I suggest you work through the patterns in the order presented here, but if you prefer to take them in a different sequence, that will be all right.

SECTION ONE – THE BASIC PATTERNS

PATTERN ONE: MOTIVATIONAL LEVEL

It is essential to have a high level of motivation to achieve weight loss, and all the exercises in this book are designed to enhance your motivation levels.

If your motivation level is naturally high, you will find it easier to put all these things into practice and you may well already be well on the way to achieving the results you want. If your natural motivation level tends to be lower, you may find you need more support in achieving results. If this is the case, when you do the exercises be sure to make your mental images and sounds really strong and be sure to do the exercises to enhance feelings. The more you do this, the easier you will find it to keep yourself motivated.

If your inclination is to do things with other people, then you can ask other people to help keep you motivated to stay on your programme. Recognizing your need for external support will be useful, as you will then know how helpful the support of others will be to you.

So it is important for you to keep in mind your motivational level so that you can maximize your efforts and keep following the steps you have chosen to pursue.

PATTERN TWO: PREFERENCE FOR THINKING OR TAKING ACTION

These patterns are linked and, in the context of weight loss, are both important. Some people really like thinking at length about things before they do them, whereas others like to just jump in and have a go. As the title of this book implies, thinking is vital when losing weight, but taking action is vital too, otherwise nothing is achieved.

If your natural inclination is to just think, you may find you have lots of good ideas that never get put into action. And if your natural inclination is to act first and think later, you may find you are always trying out new things without being certain they are going to get you where you want to be.

So, in this case, thinking and acting are *both* important. And, as you go through the exercises which follow, notice whether your natural preference is for thought or action. If it is for thought aim to balance it with action, and if it is action aim to think a little more before starting out. This may sound obvious, but paying attention to both these aspects is really important if you are to succeed. So, think *and then* act, and you will get results.

PATTERN THREE: TIME

This is an interesting pattern. Some people spend a good deal of time thinking about the past, others think a lot about the future and some are absolutely rooted in the present.

When you want to lose weight, it is important to have a strong sense of the future as you want it to be, otherwise you are likely never to get there. However, there are also some advantages to thinking about the past and the present.

In the past you were slimmer, even if it was a long time ago. So keeping the past in mind can be helpful in reminding you that you do have that potential. It is also important to remember the present. If you spend all your time *thinking* about the future or the past, you may forget to *do* those things which need to be done *now*.

So being able to keep past, present and future – and especially the future – in mind is important to you. When you go through the following exercises, do remember to practise thinking about all these times and, if you have difficulty in thinking about the future and creating a really compelling sense of how you can be, it is worth taking time to develop your skills in making the future real. Have another look at chapter 2 where I told you about some exercises to develop your mental skills and apply these to doing the following:

- picturing yourself in the future, as you would like to be
- being really clear about your future image of yourself; making it bright, clear and colourful
- really seeing the detail of how that 'future you' looks; your face, your figure, your expression, your hair, your movement and so on
- then 'stepping into' this image and really feeling what the future will be like when you look like your image

As long as the future image you are making is realistic, this process of putting it in your mind will really work to make it come true.

PATTERN FOUR: USING DIFFERENT SENSES

This pattern is to do with the extent to which you use your different senses. It may be that you rely on *visual* stimulation to motivate you to do things, it may be that you need to *hear* things that support your efforts, or it may be that you just need to *feel* right to start achieving.

Whatever your own preferences are, you will find they are catered for in the exercises which follow. And you have two choices as to how you use this knowledge. First you can choose to use your preferred senses even more, as you know they work for you already. So if you know you need to see things before doing them (if for example you need to see the food in a restaurant before knowing what to select), you can choose those exercises which show you how to visualize success. Secondly, you could choose to develop those senses which you do not use to such a great extent, so that they can contribute more than they do at present to your success. So if you do not rely on your feelings much, you could work on acknowledging your feelings more and becoming more aware of what you feel and how you would like to feel instead, if your present feelings are not supporting what you want to achieve.

It is up to you, but I would suggest following the second choice, as enhancing all your senses will give you a more rounded experience and more ways of helping your programme along.

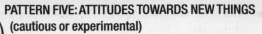

PATTERN FIVE: ATTITUDES TOWARDS NEW THINGS (cautious or experimental)

This is a useful pattern to understand, as it provides you with information on your basic approach to new things. If your pattern is that of caution, you are likely to need to know that ideas have been well tried and tested before you use them. This means that when following a weight- control programme, it will be helpful for you to know that, for example, guidelines on healthy eating are internationally recognized and that exercise has proven medical benefits. If your pattern is experimentation, you probably enjoy trying out new things. This means that you can vary your programme, incorporating new ideas as you come across them. You will probably also be very interested in the ideas about how to use your mind, as they may well be new to you, even though they have already had major effects in helping many people achieve success.

SECTION TWO – THE EXPLORATORY PATTERNS

Having covered the first five patterns, you will now have a good idea of how they can affect the ways in which you can approach losing weight. Let's move on now to the next set of patterns and explore these in more detail.

I have split each pattern into its separate categories – based on the A, B, C and D answers you gave in the tests in chapter 3 – and you will find guidance for them all. For each of the pattern elements, you will find ideas on the steps to take to:

- set effective goals
- think and feel purposeful

- behave in ways which will help move you towards your goals
- maintain positive beliefs about yourself and your progress

When I ask you to do an exercise which involves thinking creatively, it will help if you get into a relaxed state by sitting or lying down and, if it helps, playing yourself some calming music. Making sure you find time for yourself to go through these exercises will really help keep you on track and make your programme a success.

Remember, too, that if you need any more practice at the techniques I have told you about, wherever you see a diagram next to any part of an exercise, you can turn back to the same diagram in an earlier part of the book to find more about how to do that kind of technique.

And finally, remember that you will have your own unique combination of patterns so, as you go through each one, remember to think about the guidance as a whole, rather than simply as isolated elements. By the time you have reached the end of pattern ten you will have a good deal of information about what you can do to achieve results and consequently will be able to understand much more about what motivates you as a unique individual.

PATTERN SIX: SELF RELIANCE (EXTERNAL)

If you are in this category, you are probably very sensitive to how other people think and you probably need to know what others think about you, or about things you are considering doing, before making up your mind about them. You will probably not start a new programme without knowing that it has been approved by others and you are likely to get on better

95

when you get good feedback from others about your progress.

If this sounds like you, have a go at the following.

GOALS

If you are external, your goals will need to be ones that you know have been recognized by others as achievable; you may also need to know that other people have already achieved similar things. You will probably prefer to have outside confirmation that you are doing well and your motivation levels may be raised when others give you encouragement. So choose goals which involve other people's support, such as joining a class where you can get feedback on your progress, or going shopping with a friend, and you will do well.

THOUGHTS

Your mind is the key to getting results. External people often have things in their minds which involve other people. For example, they may imagine people making comments about them; they may picture themselves at social events where people react to them in particular ways; they may feel bad if they think others are being critical or making fun of them. So what can you do to make your mind help you rather than hold you back? Find a quiet place and have a go at the following exercises. It does not matter how long you take to do them and you will find them easier the more you practise.

- Picture yourself in a group of people, looking the way you would like to look. See the other people looking at you in an admiring way. Make this picture very big, bright and clear. See the people coming towards you with friendly smiles. Visualize what it will be like to be accepted as a member of the group.

- Think about the scene you have just imagined. Now hear the people's voices as they speak to you. Listen to them complimenting you on how successful you have been in losing weight. In your mind, make the voices sound pleasant and welcoming. Hear these voices as if there are people all round you, saying positive things. Make the voices very clear. Listen to the different voice tones from the different people as they speak.

- Hear your own voice in your head, telling you how well you are doing. Make it sound positive. Make it as loud as you need, so you are sure it is giving you a positive message – as if you were hearing someone else tell you those things.

- Imagine a food you have been tempted by in the past. Remember its smell and its taste. Now imagine someone who you know is well informed about food telling you that you should eat something different instead. As you hear the voice, imagine the smell and taste of the other food and imagine yourself eating it. As you taste the food in your mouth, hear the person who suggested it saying 'Well done' for making that choice.

FEELINGS

Allow yourself to project into the future and think about what kind of feeling you would like to have as you make progress. For example, how about the feeling of being encouraged by your friends. Now think back to a time in the past when you were encouraged by someone and, as you re-experience that occasion in your mind, allow yourself to have the sense of what you saw, what you heard and how you felt at that time. Associate that feeling with a signal, such as touching your earlobe. Really allow the feeling and the signal to become connected. Now think about a time in the future, when it will be really useful to feel that you are being encouraged and, as you think of that time, give yourself the signal (touching your earlobe) again. In this way, the signal will become associated in your mind with that feeling, and you will be able to create, or strengthen, the feeling at will. Think up as many different signals as you like for as many different feelings as you like so you can draw upon them whenever you need to keep yourself on track.

BEHAVIOUR

Because you think other people's opinions are important, you are more likely to choose behaviour which is approved of by others, or which will lead to good feedback from other people. How about the following?

- Phone a friend every few days to talk about how you are getting on.
- Follow the healthy eating guidelines which the health bodies have said are good for everyone.
- Check your exercise progress with a fitness professional from time to time.
- Ask your closest friend or relative to tell you that you are doing well when you achieve one of your goals.
- Spend time with people you know will be positive rather than negative about your programme.

By doing these things which include other people, you will be more comfortable with your programme and more certain of getting the support you need to continue.

BELIEFS

Changing beliefs is easier when you have had an experience which gives you a different perspective on things. For example, if you think other people are critical of you but then find out they are impressed with what you have done, you may well change your beliefs about how they react to you.

An excellent way of creating new beliefs is by repeating positive things to yourself on a regular basis. You might choose to say these things out loud, to hear them in your head or to put them up as posters on the wall and read them every time you go past. How about the following?

- If it is possible for them it is possible for me.
- As I achieve my goals, people can see how well I am doing.
- I am getting all the support I need.
- I can ask for help whenever I need it.
- I am capable of all the things people tell me I can do.

You can of course add to this list, or get your friends to suggest phrases which you might use – there are a lot to choose from and you will find it really helpful.

We have now covered a range of things you can do to keep on track; now you can make a start, knowing that support and encouragement is available for what you are doing.

PATTERN SIX: SELF-RELIANCE (INTERNAL)

If you are in this category, you will probably be very good at deciding things for yourself. You will probably have clear standards of your own for things and know when things are going well or badly without others having to tell you or give you feedback.

99

You are likely to be self-motivated and not need a push from others to get started. If this describes you, have a go at the following exercises.

GOALS
When setting goals, you will need to find things you can be in control of. It will be important to you to make the decisions about when to start and stop activities, for example whether to walk to work, what to eat for breakfast and where to shop, and you will want to decide for yourself how well you are doing. As long as you can be in charge, you are likely to do well. So choose goals which you know are right for you, or which you can be in control of; really think about what it is that you want and then pursue it with all your energy. By doing this, you will be certain to be better motivated to achieve results.

THOUGHTS
As a person who is good at deciding things for yourself, you can use your mind to help you do things the way you want. So you can create thoughts which include doing things in your own way; for example:

- Picture yourself in a supermarket deciding to buy healthy foods and rejecting the ones which will set your programme back. Really make the image of this clear, bright, large and appealing. See yourself exactly as you would be; notice what you would be wearing, how quickly or slowly you would be moving, which parts of the supermarket you would be walking up and down. See the products on the shelves, noticing the colours and shapes of the items. Hear the sound of the other people moving about and talking. Feel the air and notice how cool it is around the chilled products. Notice the smell of the fresh fruit and vegetables. Now, as you see yourself selecting one of the healthy items, imagine you are 'stepping into' your body in the mental image you have created and really feel yourself stretching out for the item and putting it in your basket; notice how good it makes you feel to have chosen something which will really help your programme. Now see yourself at home, unpacking your purchases and then preparing your meal. Hear the sounds you make as you move around the kitchen putting things together. Imagine how the food will look and smell as you prepare it. Now imagine the taste of the food as you eat it, knowing you have made a good choice which will contribute to your programme.

- In your mind, tell yourself you are going to stick to your programme. Make your voice very positive and encouraging. Hear the exact words you are saying, each one very clear and distinct. Hear yourself say exactly what you need to do to make it work. Give yourself some praise for what you are doing.

- In your mind, hear some people you know saying how easily you seem to control what you eat. Imagine them telling you how well you are doing. Make their voices very close to you and, as you hear their voices, picture them in your mind, looking encouraging and pleased for you.

Make all these mental images and sounds as powerful and compelling as possible. Make the pictures very clear and bright and see them close up. Make the sound of your own voice positive and decisive. Make the sounds of other people's voices admiring and complimentary. Really experience the feelings that these mental sounds and images give you; your mind will hold onto them and remind you of them as you go along.

FEELINGS

We have talked about how your mind can produce images and sounds which lead you into positive feelings. You can also create more positive feelings by doing the next exercise.

Allow yourself to project into the future and decide what kind of feelings would help you keep to your programme. As an example, take the feeling of determination. Think back to a time in the past when you felt really determined to achieve something. It does not matter how small that thing was, the important thing is that you really followed it through.

As you remember that time, let the feelings you had then come back to you now. Do this by remembering where you were, what you could see, what you could hear and how you felt. As soon as you re-experience the feeling of determination, give yourself a signal, perhaps pressing your toe against the ground. As you do this, notice how the feeling and the signal link together.

Now imagine yourself in the future, at a time when you will need the feeling of determination and, still thinking about that situation, give yourself the same signal (pressing your toe against the ground) and notice how the feeling of determination comes back. You can use this technique any time you need to create or re-inforce the feeling you have

102

selected. And if you want an additional feeling, as well as determination, just repeat the process, choosing a different signal for each additional feeling you choose.

BEHAVIOUR

As you are good at making decisions for yourself, the behaviour changes you will need are ones which mean you can decide exactly what to do. How about some of the following?

- going out for a walk when you feel like doing so
- planning your meals a week in advance so you know what you will be eating each day
- eating those foods you know are good for you
- having a rest when you feel like it
- putting unhealthy foods away so they will not tempt you
- leaving yourself notes as reminders to keep to your plans

These are all things you can be in control of and manage for yourself. How many other things can you think of that you can be in charge of yourself? Remember that if you are in situations where you feel out of control you may tend to get frustrated or demotivated, so make sure you keep on track by giving yourself things to do which will really keep *you* in the driving seat.

BELIEFS

To do well at your programme, it will help if you convince yourself that you will succeed. An excellent and simple way of doing this is to repeat things to yourself, either in your head or out loud (or you can pin them up on the wall and read them each time you go past).

103

Because you like being in control of your world, you may find the following useful, or you can choose any other statements which you feel appeal to you more:

- I am looking after myself well.
- I am capable of choosing exactly what to eat to help me achieve my goals.
- I am able to decide exactly how much exercise to take each day.
- I am making a real contribution to my future life.
- I am the only one who is capable of managing my weight.

These are some of the things you can do to ensure your programme is a success. Using your mind effectively is a great support to you; practise and persevere and you will be able to create the changes you seek.

PATTERN SEVEN: SOCIABILITY (INTRAPERSONAL)
If you are in this category you probably like to do things on your own. You function best when you can get on with things without being interrupted. You may sometimes find it frustrating having to do things with others, as you cannot go at your own pace. You need time and space to 'do your own thing'.

If this sounds like you, have a go at the following.

GOALS

When setting your goals, you need to find things which you can do on your own. You will work best if you have time alone to concentrate and take things at your own pace. So remember to set goals which allow you to do things in your own way, such as cooking a meal the way you like or going for a walk at your own pace.

THOUGHTS

As a person who likes doing things alone, you can use your mind to help you create a future where you are doing things the way you like. You will already have done the 'present state' part of this process in chapter 4 and seen if there are any thoughts in your mind which are negative. If there are, you can use your mind to give you images and sounds which will support what you wish to do. Some examples of positive thoughts are the following.

- See yourself doing one of the activities you have chosen; picture yourself on your own and enjoying the time you are spending by yourself. Really see yourself in detail; notice the 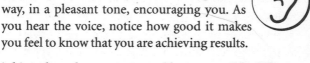 expression on your face and notice the way you are sitting, standing or moving. Once you have seen the image, imagine 'stepping into' it and really feeling the experience. Notice if there are any sounds associated with the activity and, if there are, hear them in your head. Also notice any other features of the environment in which you are doing the activity (for example with swimming there is a typical smell of chlorine; with walking you may notice the feel of the air on your face or the sun on your back). Really experience the activity as if you were there.
- Tell yourself (in your mind) that you are making good progress; hear your voice in a positive way, in a pleasant tone, encouraging you. As you hear the voice, notice how good it makes you feel to know that you are achieving results.

Thinking about how you can tackle any possible difficulties which could arise is also helpful. By spending time thinking about these, you can be prepared for them and work out the best ways of dealing with them. This will prevent you from becoming stressed and you will be less likely to succumb to food as a remedy for being under pressure.

Make all your mental images and sounds as attractive as you can. Play around with making the pictures bigger, brighter and more colourful. Really see yourself doing well. Make your voice more and more positive and encouraging, so you really believe what it says.

FEELINGS

Allow yourself to project into the future and think about what kind of feeling would be useful in supporting your programme. Perhaps it will be a feeling of achievement. Now remember a time when you really felt you had achieved something and, thinking back to the memory of that time, give yourself a signal (perhaps scratching the side of your nose gently) to remind you of that feeling. Now, as you think about the future, give yourself the signal (scratching your nose) and, at the same time, imagine yourself feeling, again, that you are really achieving results in that future time.

BEHAVIOUR

As you like doing things on your own, you will need to find some activities which you can do by yourself. There are lots to choose from and the following will give you a few ideas; you can then add to the list as you think of more things.

- **Making time for yourself.** Setting aside some time each day to follow your programme will give you the opportunity to make real progress. Some of the things you can do in this time include:

- relaxing and getting into a positive state
- having a warm bath with soothing or energizing oils, washing your hair, putting on nice clothes or make-up so you look good – all these things can give you a boost and make you feel better about yourself during the day
- planning what you will do during the day or on the following day

- **Working out.** Here are some active things you can do to assist your programme:

  - going for a brisk walk
  - climbing stairs instead of taking a lift
  - getting off a bus or train one stop early to walk the rest of your journey
  - putting on an exercise video or a dance tape or CD at home and exercising to it
  - doing your housework faster than usual to use up more energy
  - using household objects to do exercises with, such as lifting cans of food or stepping on and off the first step of your staircase (please check on how to do such exercises before beginning; the Useful Addresses section will give you some ideas on how to get this advice)

You may think of other things you can do and add them to the above lists for yourself.

BELIEFS
To help strengthen your beliefs about what is possible for you to achieve you might like to use statements

which you can say to yourself to reinforce your performance. You can do this either by saying the things out loud or by saying them to yourself, in your head. Alternatively, you could put them on posters on the wall and read them each time you go by. Here are some suggestions for you (and you will notice they are all stated in the present – as if they are happening now).

- I am managing my weight.
- I am capable of achieving my goals.
- I am enjoying getting closer to the results I want.
- I am able to say 'No' to unhealthy food.
- I am able to exercise comfortably and enjoyably.

As you get into the habit of saying these things, your mind will get into the habit of believing them. And once your mind does, you will too.

PATTERN SEVEN: SOCIABILITY (INTERPERSONAL)

If you are in this category you probably prefer to do things in the company of others. You are likely to enjoy the stimulation of being with other people and are best motivated when others are around to give you help and support.

If this sounds like you, have a go at the following.

GOALS

You will need to set goals which include others in some way – for example, taking exercise in classes with others, having a friend to keep you on track or getting your family to support what you are doing. Choose goals which have a social element to them and where you are able to discuss your activities and do things with other people.

THOUGHTS

As a person who likes to do things with others, you can use your thoughts to create situations where you are with other people and things are going well. Have a go at the following exercises.

- Picture yourself at an exercise class or going for a walk with friends. Really see yourself in that situation, making your mental image clear, bright, large and colourful. See the detail of what you are doing; notice how you are moving, what expression you have on your face, how the other people are looking, and so on. Include sounds in your thoughts; so you might hear the sound of your feet as you walk along or as you step on and off equipment. You might hear the sound of music being played in the class. You might hear your friends' voices as they talk to you. And notice any physical sensations, such as the clothes you are wearing, the temperature of the air and so on. As you imagine this experience, put yourself in the picture and really imagine how it feels to be there. Really experience it as if it were happening right now. This will give your mind the idea that the event has taken place and will draw you towards it. It will also be more motivating to know that you can do these things in the company of your friends.

- Imagine going shopping with a friend for some clothes to wear while exercising. Hear yourselves chatting about the things you see and deciding what to buy. Be aware of enjoying the company and feeling really pleased with your purchases.

- See yourself having a meal out with friends. Imagine

the table and chairs and where everyone will be sitting. See their faces and hear their voices. See the place settings and the table covering. Now imagine the menu and see the different items on it. See how the healthier foods seem to stand out from the menu, as if they were drawing your attention to them. Picture yourself selecting one of those healthy options and see it coming to the table, looking really inviting. Imagine the taste and smell of the food you have selected. Imagine being in that image now, and really imagine eating that food and enjoying its taste and the sensation of it in your mouth. Enjoy the experience of being with your friends and still being able to choose, and enjoy, the food which will help your programme.

FEELINGS

Allow yourself to project into the future and think about what kind of feeling would be useful in supporting your programme. Maybe it will be a feeling of enjoyment at sharing an activity with your friends. Now remember a time when you did enjoy being in the company of friends and remember where you were, what you could see, what you could hear and how you felt. As soon as you have recreated that event, and remember the feeling of enjoyment, give yourself a signal, for example blinking your eyes quickly three times, and associate the signal with that feeling. Now think about the future and, as you give yourself that signal (blinking quickly) again, you can bring back that positive feeling and project it into the future, becoming aware that you can really have that feeling of enjoyment whenever you choose.

BEHAVIOUR

As you like doing things with others, you will need to find some activities which involve other people. There are lots you can select and here are some of them; you can also choose your own in addition to these.

- joining an exercise class
- sharing a healthy meal with friends
- walking each lunchtime with a workmate
- finding a friend who can meet you once a week and share your experience of the past few days
- setting up a local group to meet and support each other while you lose weight
- involving others in your programme – for example, making sure your family eat healthily too by cooking meals for everyone with low-fat ingredients and plenty of fresh fruit and vegetables; encouraging your children to exercise more by taking them for walks (especially if you have a dog which needs exercising), or by leaving the car at home for very short trips; or taking out a family membership to a leisure centre, where everyone can take part in the activities on offer

Doing some of these things will help keep you motivated and you will be able to enjoy the company of your friends as well as keeping to your plan.

BELIEFS

To help give you positive beliefs about what you can achieve, it is really useful to say things to yourself which support your activities. You can either say these out loud, say them in your head or put them on posters on the wall and read them to yourself each time you go past. How about the following?

111

- I am going to my exercise class regularly.
- I am telling people how well I am doing.
- I can see myself at social events looking good.
- I am avoiding being tempted by others into things I do not want.
- I am feeling happy about sharing my experiences with friends.

As you can see, you should make all these statements as if they are happening right now; this works much better than simply saying you are going to do something in the future. Maybe you can add other sayings of your own, or get your friends to help you think up more.

PATTERN EIGHT: DIRECTION OF MOTIVATION (TOWARDS)

If you are in this category, you are likely to be motivated by achieving goals. You find targets stimulating and are aware of things you want to work towards. You may well be so focused on your goals that you fail to see any obstacles in the way, which can be good, in that you are determined to succeed, but at the same time can cause problems if you do not anticipate things which need to be tackled on the way. So when you set yourself goals, be aware of your natural tendency to strive for things and just be realistic in the targets you set for yourself.

GOALS
You are likely to work best towards goals when they are things you really wish to achieve. The clearer and more focused you can make your goals, the easier they will be for you to achieve.

THOUGHTS

You should be able to allow your mind to help you achieve results, as you will be able to keep your objectives in mind. How about the following to keep you motivated?

- Picture each of your goals in your mind, in turn. Really get a clear image of what it is that you want to achieve. See yourself the way you would like to be and make the image bright and appealing. See as much detail as you can put into it. Now imagine stepping into that image and feel what it would be like to be that way. Imagine how your body would feel and how it would move. Hear the sound of your voice as you tell people what you have achieved. Allow your mind to create this image of the new you.

- In your mind, hear other people saying how good you are at working towards your goals. Hear their voices sounding lively and praising you. Notice how encouraged you can feel when you hear them speaking this way.

- In your mind, tell yourself to keep on track and go for your goals. Make your voice really positive and encouraging.

You can create whatever thoughts you want in your mind and the stronger the images and sounds, the more they are likely to motivate you to achieve results.

FEELINGS

Now, allow your mind to project you into the future and notice what kind of feeling it would be useful to have when you are working towards your goals. Perhaps a good feeling would be persistence;

keeping on track, knowing you are going for something worthwhile. Now think back to a time in the past when you really were persistent about something – not necessarily something connected with weight. Allow yourself to think back to that time and remember where you were and what you could see and hear, and how you felt. As you get the feeling of persistence back, give yourself a signal (such as tapping your foot up and down). As you do this, notice that the signal and the feeling become interconnected and reinforce each other. Now think to a time in the future when it will be important to you to retain that persistence and, as you do so, give yourself the signal (tapping your foot) again. Notice how the feeling of persistence comes back when you use the signal. You can use this technique any time in the future when you need an additional boost.

BEHAVIOUR

As someone who is focused on goals, your behaviour needs to be goal-related for you to be successful. So how about some of the following things to do?

- Plan in advance exactly what you need to achieve.
- Set yourself short- , medium- and long-term goals.
- Have daily and weekly goals, eg what meals you will eat and what exercise you will take.
- Tell people about your goals, or remind yourself about them regularly to keep them in your mind.

BELIEFS

It is useful to repeat certain things to yourself to keep yourself motivated. You can do this either by saying them out loud or by repeating them to yourself in your head. Alternatively, you could put them on posters on the wall and read them each time you go past. Some of the things you might tell yourself are:

- I am succeeding in achieving my goals.
- I am clear about what I have to achieve.
- I know I can keep to my chosen path.

As you repeat the sayings, your mind comes to believe them and, when your mind does, so will you.

PATTERN EIGHT: DIRECTION OF MOTIVATION (AWAY FROM)

If you are in this category, you probably naturally avoid things which cause problems and only take action when the present state has become intolerable. Instead of aiming for a goal because it is what you want, you may aim for it because it helps you avoid something else. Let me give you an example. Suppose you spend a lot of time cleaning your house. It may be that you do it because you really enjoy living in a house which looks immaculate – this is 'towards' behaviour; you are doing it for its own sake, because that is the result you want. However, you might spend time cleaning your house because you do not want visitors to think it looks dirty or untidy. In this case you would not be keeping it clean simply because you wanted it that way, but because of the consequences of *not* cleaning it. So, if you are in this category – away from – you are likely to be motivated by getting away from things you do not like.

So what does this mean in relation to slimming? It means that you will be best motivated to keep to your programme because of what will happen if you do not. And that could include being unfit and suffering from problems with mobility or breathlessness; it could include criticism from other people or it could include not being able to buy clothes in the styles you want.

How does this knowledge affect your programme? Let us take it one element at a time.

GOALS

When setting yourself goals you should think of what will happen if you do not achieve them. So, if you do not eat a healthy diet, what will happen? If you do not exercise twice a week, what will happen? And if there is no obvious 'downside' then you may need to invent one to keep yourself motivated.

THOUGHTS

Your mind will be best able to help you if you put thoughts into it about what will happen if you continue to be overweight. Some of the following could work for you.

- Picture yourself in a year's time weighing even more than you do now. See this image very clearly, in close-up, with lots of detail. Now imagine how your body would feel at that weight. Seeing and feeling the consequences of continuing the way you are should act to keep you on track.
- In your mind, hear other people being critical of you, or saying you look unfit or flabby. Again, make these imaginary voices loud and clear so that you can really hear them distinctly. This should help motivate you to avoid such comments.
- Hear your own voice in your head saying that if you do not keep to the programme you will be miserable and look and feel unhealthy.
  - Hear your own voice telling you that you are doing so well in overcoming all the difficulties and obstacles you felt were in your way in the past.

All these things will keep you on track.

FEELINGS

Take a moment to let your mind come up with a feeling which would be useful to you in your programme. As you are motivated by moving away from things, this might be the feeling of being bloated and uncomfortable. Think back to a time when you actually felt like that; in your mind, remember the occasion and think back to where you were, what you could see at the time, what you could hear and how you felt. As you get that feeling back, give yourself a signal (possibly gently biting the tip of your tongue). Really make a connection between the signal and the feelings. Now think of a time in the future when it would be useful for you to have that feeling again, to warn you off eating the wrong kinds of food or making excuses for not exercising. As you think of that future time, give yourself the signal again (biting your tongue) and notice how the feeling of discomfort returns. Use this triggering device at any time, when you want to remind yourself how bad you will feel if you do not continue with your programme.

BEHAVIOUR

Keeping your motivation pattern in mind, now turn your attention to the things you can do to keep your programme going. How about some of the following?

- In food shops, as soon as you find yourself near the counters for high-fat, sweet things, move away from them, remembering how they will make you feel and look.
- Avoid travelling to work by car wherever possible; walk or cycle instead.
- Stop snacking and give yourself well-balanced meals instead of constant nibbles.

117

- Look in mirrors while shopping so you see what you need to change about yourself.

BELIEFS

It has been shown that repeating certain things to yourself on a regular basis helps keep you motivated. You can either say things to yourself out loud or do it in your head. Or you can put up posters on your wall and then read them each time you pass. How about some of the following things to say to yourself?

- I am avoiding all the things which used to tempt me.
- I am getting away from my old eating habits.
- I am sitting around the house less.
- I am overcoming the negative thoughts I used to have.

Saying this kind of thing to yourself will keep it in your mind and, if your mind believes it, you will do so too.

PATTERN NINE: DEGREE OF FLEXIBILITY (RULES)

If you are in this category, you probably feel most comfortable when you know exactly what has to be done. You like to have a system for doing things and you probably think about what is the 'right way' to do things. You may not like things to be haphazard because you work best when they are orderly and predictable.

If this sounds like you, have a go at the following.

GOALS

When setting your goals you will need to be careful to break them down into stages which are logical and well structured. You can think out how the different aspects of your programme fit together and work towards doing the right thing for you. Remember to give yourself orderly steps to take to achieve results and put things in your programme which are systematic and well organized, such as a regular time to exercise, set times for meals or a weekly meal plan with regular rotations of food items.

Because it is important for you to know the right way of approaching a weight-loss programme, you can rest assured that, in following the guidelines in this book, you will be well on the way to success.

THOUGHTS

You can use your mind to help with your programme. The best way will be for you to work through what you have to do in a systematic way. So, you might like to think about the following.

- Picture what you are going to do; see a plan of action in your mind. As you look at it, notice the different steps you need to take and how one follows another in a logical way. Tell yourself that it is right for you to follow this programme and hear your voice sounding clear and concise.
- See yourself working methodically through the steps you have laid down. First, get a good mental image of the action you will need to take and then imagine 'stepping into' the mental image and get a feel for what it will actually be like to do those things. Really get the feeling of going about your programme in an organized and well-thought-out manner.
- In your mind, hear other people saying how well you are doing. Hear them complimenting you on following your programme so

methodically. Make the voices clear and loud enough to let you know that they really mean what they are saying.

FEELINGS

In your mind, allow yourself to project into the future and think of how you would like to feel as you work through your programme. Perhaps a good feeling would be confidence in having chosen the right programme. Now, think back to a time in the past when you did feel really confident that you had chosen a correct course of action for something – it does not have to be related to weight control. Now think back to that time and remember where you were, how the place looked, any sounds you could hear and any physical sensation you had at that time. As you get the feeling back, give yourself a signal, for example pressing the thumb and forefinger of one hand together. As you do this, allow the signal to become associated with the feeling. Now, think of a time in the future when you will need to feel really confident that you have chosen the right approach to losing weight. Give yourself the signal (pressing thumb and finger together) and notice how confident you can feel in that future time.

BEHAVIOUR

If you like things to be orderly and systematic, you will enjoy choosing things to do which you can predict and which are organized well. You might like to have a go at some of these.

- Join an organized class.
- Schedule certain activities for the same time each day so that you will be sure to do them.

- Do your exercises correctly, using the right amount of effort and control for each.
- Make sure your meals each day are well balanced and contain the right combinations of food elements.
- Read food labels before buying to be sure they contain exactly what you need.
- Have a structured programme of exercise, so you can step it up in logical, progressive stages.

BELIEFS

To keep you going, it is worth working on the things you believe about what is possible. It has been found that by frequently repeating certain messages to yourself, your mind begins to believe they are true. You can either say these messages out loud or you can say them to yourself in your head, or you can put them up on posters and read them every time you pass. Some of the things you might find useful to say are:

- I am doing all the right things I need to succeed.
- I have a good system for controlling my weight.
- I am losing the right amount of weight each week.
- I have the ability to keep on the right track.
- I am capable of achieving my goals in a systematic way.

By making these statements sound as if they are happening right now, your mind will believe they are, and will produce ways of achieving your goals.

PATTERN NINE: DEGREE OF FLEXIBILITY (OPTIONS)

If you are in this category, you will probably like to have lots of different ways of doing things. You may well get bored with following the same procedures all the time and seek variety and choice.

121

Options people like to be able to vary what they do and to come up with lots of ideas for how they do things.

If this sounds like you, have a go at the following.

GOALS

When setting goals, it is worth remembering that you may get bored if things stay the same for too long, so keep variety in what you set out to do. For example, instead of saying you will go for a walk each day, think about walking one day and jogging another, or walking one day and going swimming the next, or walking for one day each week and then changing to another activity. Similarly with food, you might choose to have hot food one day and cold the next, or Italian meals for one week and then Indian. The choice is up to you.

THOUGHTS

You can get your mind to help you become sufficiently stimulated by the range of thoughts you have. So, how about considering these possibilities.

- Picture yourself going shopping for food and noticing all the different kinds of foods on offer. See the variety available. Imagine looking at the fruit and vegetable counter, or at the fresh fish section. Really picture those foods which you can have in your programme and see their shapes and colours in real detail. Now imagine picking up some of the foods, for example an orange, some broccoli or a bunch of grapes. Feel their texture and their weight. Smell their scent. Notice how it feels being able to have so many options in choosing a healthy menu.

- In your mind, listen to some of the things other people have said about the ways in which they lose weight. Maybe one has an exercise routine which contains some things you could do too. Perhaps one makes an excellent soup out of fresh ingredients. Possibly one is very good at planning out what to do. Listen to the voices in your mind, making them sound enthusiastic and noticing the variety in voice tones and ways of speaking. Again, you can become aware of how many options there are for you to consider.

- Hear your own voice, in your mind, running through how you will approach your own programme. Listen to what you will be doing in the first week, the second week and so on. Check that there is enough variety for you to feel really motivated by it.

FEELINGS

Now allow yourself to project into the future and think about what kind of feeing would be helpful in keeping you motivated. Maybe a good feeling would be excitement at the variety of choices open to you. So think back to a time in the past when you did feel excited about the choices you had open to you. (And if you cannot remember such a time, just think back to any time you felt really excited about anything.) In your mind, remember the experience and picture where you were and what you could see, what you could hear and how you felt. As soon as you get back that feeling of excitement, give yourself a signal, such as tapping your elbow with the fingers of one hand. Really experience how the signal and the feelings seem to link together.

Now think about a time in the future when it will be helpful for you to feel excited about your programme options and give yourself the signal

123

(tapping your elbow) again. As you do so, notice how you can feel really excited in that future time.

BEHAVIOUR

As you like choices, it will be important to you to have real variety and options in your programme. How about some of these to start with?

- Plan to do a different activity each week.
- Only plan one week's menus and leave the following week's to nearer the time.
- Buy foods in season, so that you get different things to eat at different times.
- Walk as often as possible rather than using public transport or driving, taking as many different routes as you can find.
- If you use a gym, vary the order in which you use the equipment, so it is always new and interesting.
- Experiment with new techniques and approaches which are suitable for your programme.

BELIEFS

It has been shown to be really useful to repeat to yourself certain things which can add to your motivation. You can say these things out loud or to yourself in your head, or you can put them on posters and pin them up on the wall so you can read them when you go past. You might like to use the following, or to make up others of your own; you can change the things you say from time to time, but do make sure you keep to the same ones for at least a couple of weeks before changing.

- I am able to do well at all the different aspects of my programme.

124

- I can choose my meals to fit in with my changing weight loss.
- I have the ability to select activities which will work well for me.

As you repeat these things, your mind begins to believe them and, once your mind believes them, you can too.

PATTERN TEN: NEED FOR DETAIL (SPECIFIC)

If you are in this category, you probably like to know exactly where you are, what you have to do and how to do it. You enjoy having detailed explanations and knowing exactly what you are involved in. This means that before you start a programme you will enjoy knowing exactly what it entails and having instructions and clear guidance about what you have to do.

If this sounds like you, have a go at the following.

GOALS

When setting goals, they need to be sufficiently detailed for you to understand and keep to. So specify them clearly and explicitly. Put as much detail as you need to work with them; for example 'I will buy fresh vegetables regularly – at least two different kinds each day, some green and some red, and eat at least one a day uncooked.'

THOUGHTS

Your mind can help you, but it is likely to need you to provide it with the detail to do so. How about the following as ideas for managing your mind?

- Picture yourself working towards one of your goals. Really see what you would be doing. This might be cooking a healthy meal, for example. In this case, you would need to picture

125

yourself in your kitchen; see the room and the furniture and the equipment. Watch yourself getting all the utensils together. See yourself switching on the oven, or turning on the hot plates. See yourself moving around and doing all the things you need in order to prepare the meal. Now imagine 'stepping into' the image you are seeing, and really feel what it will be like making that meal. Feel the implements in your hands; smell the food as it is prepared, perhaps get a taste of any of the things you need to test – for example whether there is enough seasoning in the food. Listen to the sounds you make as you cook the food; perhaps stirring ingredients in a saucepan, or pouring liquid into a container. As you do this, the detail will bring the scene to life and will really motivate you to turn it into reality.

- In your mind hear other people telling you how well you are doing to change from how you were. Really hear their voices loudly and clearly. Hear exactly what they are saying to you and notice how good it makes you feel to know you are doing exactly what you need to achieve results.

- In your mind, hear your own voice telling you exactly what you need to do to make progress . Make your voice really positive and certain that you are able to make those detailed changes you need in order to move forward.

FEELINGS

Allow your mind to take you into the future and let you know what kind of feeling would be useful in helping you achieve results. Maybe that feeling would be one of pleasure at having got all the details right. Now think back to a time in the past when you really did get all the details of something right, not necessarily anything to do with your weight. Now, as you think back to that time, remember where you were and what you could see and hear at that time; also remember exactly how you felt. As you do this, give yourself a signal, for example bringing your teeth together briefly. Really associate the signal with the feeling of pleasure at getting things right. Now think about a time in the future when it would be really useful to feel you had got the detail right in your programme. As you think of that time, give yourself the signal (teeth together) and notice how the feeling of pleasure comes flooding back. You can be confident that whenever you need that feeling in the future you now have a way of creating it for yourself.

BEHAVIOUR

You will have realized that it is important for you to have enough detail when you are doing things, so have a go at the following, or add other activities which you feel are more appropriate for you.

- Make a really explicit plan of what you are going to do in your programme. Put in what you will be doing each day. (*See* the next chapter for more information on the process of planning.)
- Sort out your menus for the next week. Work out exactly what you will be having to eat and what ingredients you need to buy. Make a list of them all. (You will find more information on lists in the next chapter.)
- If you use exercise equipment, find out exactly what effect each piece of equipment has on your body.

There should be charts next to each one; do read them and be sure you understand exactly how they work.

BELIEFS

It is important to let your mind realize that you can do well. It has been found that by repeating certain things to yourself on a regular basis, your mind listens and takes in what you say. You can do this by saying things out loud or in your head, or you can put the things down on posters and pin them to the wall, so you can read them each time you pass by.

Some of the things you might like to repeat are:

- I am following my programme, right down to the last detail.
- I am capable of doing exactly what I need to do.
- Every part of my programme is working well.
- I know exactly what I need to eat to keep healthy and lose weight.

The more you repeat these things the more your mind will believe them; and when your mind believes them, you will too.

PATTERN TEN: NEED FOR DETAIL (GENERAL)

If you are in this category you probably like to take an overview of things. You are more comfortable with a rough outline of what to do than with a very detailed breakdown or explanation. This means you are more likely to be motivated when you can get a good sense of direction rather than a detailed route map.

What does this mean for your programme? Maybe you would like to consider some of the following ideas.

128

GOALS

You will probably get on best if you set out your goals fairly broadly, rather than being too explicit about them. For example, you might simply have a goal of trying different kinds of exercise, without knowing in advance which ones you want to try.

You will find information on goal setting elsewhere in the book (*see* page 73) and you may find the advice I have just given you a little contradictory as, in general, goal setting needs to be explicit. What I mean here is simply that you are likely to get on best if you keep your goals as open as possible, consistent with knowing what to do. Having said that, however, even though your motivational pattern is one of not wishing to specify things too clearly, you would probably get on with your programme better if you did keep your goal setting more specific. This is one of those occasions where it is really useful to have a go at extending your own patterns into new territory.

THINKING

Your mind can be of considerable help in achieving results and, with a motivational preference for generalization, you can allow your mind to do some of the following:

- Picture yourself being successful at losing weight. You do not need to specify exactly how much weight you will have lost at that time, but simply know that you are getting on well with your programme. Picture yourself doing well and create a good mental image of yourself. Notice the overall impression you would create as a slimmer person. Now, imagine how it will feel when you have reached that stage.

129

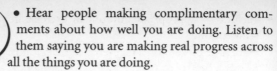

- Hear people making complimentary comments about how well you are doing. Listen to them saying you are making real progress across all the things you are doing.

- Tell yourself you are succeeding overall and can achieve the results you need.

FEELINGS

Allow your mind to project you into the future. As you do this, think of a feeling which you would find useful. Perhaps a good feeling would be an overall sense of wellbeing. Now think back to a time in the past when you felt that way. As you do this, remember where you were and what you could see and hear. Remember how you felt and, as you recall that feeling of wellbeing, give yourself a signal, maybe touching your eyebrow with your fingers. Really associate the signal with the feeling of wellbeing. Now think of a time when, in working through your programme, it would be useful to have that general sense of wellbeing and give yourself the signal. Notice how the feeling comes back to you. In the future, when you need that feeling, all you have to do is repeat the signal (touching your eyebrow) and the feeling will return.

BEHAVIOUR

Because you prefer to work with the broad picture in mind, rather than with detail, you may sometimes find it a little difficult to put in the effort you need in order to keep on track. You can have a go at the following activities, but do remember that at some stage you are likely to need to get down to detail in some respects. So do read pages 125–8 about the 'detail' pattern, as this will give you some useful information to consider.

- Include an appropriate amount of exercise in your daily routine.
- Have a balanced diet, with plenty of fresh foods.
- Monitor how you are doing on a regular basis.
- Get enough information to keep you going.

BELIEFS

Once your mind has a belief instilled in it, it will work for you in making the belief come true. It has been found that repeating certain phrases can help you change your beliefs and you might like to repeat some of the following statements for this purpose. You can do this out loud or in your head, or alternatively you could write the statements up on posters so you can read them whenever you pass by. Have a go at some of the following, or substitute others if you have different ones you would prefer.

- I am getting better at all the things I am doing.
- I am exercising as much as I need.
- I am eating healthily.
- I am making good progress towards my goals.

The more you repeat the statements, the more your mind believes them and the more your mind believes them, the more you can too.

Imagining the future

Now that you have gone through all the different motivational and preference patterns, you will have some ideas about how to take the steps you need to achieve success. Before we move on, there is one further technique which I would like you to remember. We have

131

covered it incidentally in some of the previous sections, but I believe it is helpful to refer to it again, in more detail, here.

The technique is to imagine yourself in the future, when you have achieved your goal, something we have talked about at various times in the book. I recommend that you try this exercise, no matter which of the motivational groups you placed yourself in.

You can do it with all of your goals, but just select one of them at a time. For example you might choose a goal of swimming before you go to work. Think about the time when you will have achieved that particular goal. In your mind, make an image of the goal; really see yourself the way you would like to be. Put as much detail into the mental image as you can, making it clear, bright, colourful and full of action. Now imagine 'moving into' that image so that you really experience the feeling of achievement, hearing any sounds associated with the image and feeling any physical sensations which would be associated with it.

You can do this exercise in a physical way if you prefer, by imagining seeing yourself on the other side of a room, again making the image of yourself as positive and appealing as you can. Once you have 'seen' yourself the way you would like to be, walk across the room and stand in the spot where you had seen the imaginary image of yourself. As you stand in that place, notice how it feels to be that 'future you'.

You can do this exercise on a whole range of goals and all the evidence is that this is exactly the process which really successful people use to get results, whether in sports performance, selling, negotiating, making a speech, doing the ironing or losing weight. Once your mind has a compelling positive image to work with, results just seem to follow. So create your future in your mind and you will be helping it turn into reality as well.

Achieving natural slimness

We have talked about what you can do if you fall into one or more of the categories above. There is another process, however, which cuts across all these categories and which you will find extremely helpful to know about. This is the strategy which naturally slim people follow in managing their weight. We talked about Neuro-Linguistic Programming in chapter 2; one of the features of NLP is that it was developed by analysing how very successful people achieved their results. By following this process, you will be able to use the same methods that naturally slim people use to maintain a constant weight.

People who are naturally slim seem to have an inbuilt mechanism for controlling their weight. A number of writers, including Connirae and Steve Andreas and Deepak Chopra, have explored the strategies which naturally slim people use, and I outline their findings below so that you can learn them too.

The naturally slim seem to do three things:

- **They assess how hungry they are.** This means that, before eating, they decide if they are hungry enough to eat a meal. An easy way for you to do this is to think about a scale from one to ten, with one indicating that you are not at all hungry and ten that you are extremely hungry. You then need to assess where you are on the scale each time you think of eating. If

133

you are near the bottom of the scale, ie not very hungry, you should *not* eat. Nor should you wait until you are right at the top of the scale and extremely hungry before you eat. Somewhere towards the top end is best and certainly more than half-way up. Naturally slim people do this automatically, and you can train yourself to do it too.

- **They imagine how particular foods would feel inside them.** This means that, before eating, they imagine tasting the food in their mouth and then feeling it in their stomach. If they then feel that the food would feel all right in their stomach, not just immediately but for some time afterwards as well, they eat it. If they feel that they would be bloated or uncomfortable having eaten the food, they avoid it. They may also compare the taste and feel of different foods, one after another, before deciding which one to eat. This enables them to decide on suitable and healthy foods in a restaurant, rather than simply going for one that sounds good on the menu or looks good on the trolley. They also think about the food at each bite they take, so they constantly monitor how hungry they are and how good the food seems to them. When it becomes less appealing, they stop eating. You too can do this when you eat; you only need to get into the habit of stopping to think *before* you eat. It only takes a few seconds and you will be really glad you took the time to help yourself.

- **They stop eating when they are full (actually when they are almost full – they don't wait until they have overeaten).** This means that they let their bodies tell them when they have had enough. It generally takes at least 20 minutes for your brain to get the message that your stomach is full; there is a mechanism called the 'appestat' – a kind of 'appetite thermostat' – which lets you know when you are full. So eating slowly will help you manage how much you eat. It is also a good idea to stop short of being absolutely satiated. You can always have another meal; tomorrow is another day and food will still be around.

So, to help you control your eating, have a go at these approaches. Check your hunger level, then imagine the food inside you and only eat it if you are really hungry and you know the food will feel good inside you after some time. Check each mouthful in the same way. Then stop when you have eaten enough. If you are low on the hunger scale, or the food is not appealing after you have considered it in that way, then do something other than eating. And if you are not sure when you have had enough, *stop just before you think you are full* and wait for a few minutes to allow your feelings of hunger to subside.

Some final hints

These tips also cut across all categories; they are simply techniques which most people find helpful in losing weight.

- **Use healthy cooking processes.** Avoid using a lot of fat in cooking. If you want to fry, use a spray-on oil or use water instead, which will work well for many foods, especially stir-fries.
- **Sit down to eat.** This helps you concentrate on what you are eating, so you enjoy your food and know when you have had enough. If you eat while doing

other things it can be easy to overeat, as you are not monitoring what you are eating when your concentration is elsewhere.

- **Recognize food cravings.** There is a difference between hunger and food craving. Real hunger is a signal that your body needs energy; food cravings are a desire for a particular food or type of food, even when you may not need to eat. If you have a craving for a food, you can do one or more of the following:

  - Wait until it subsides (and it will); do something to occupy your mind or body until it goes away.
  - Recognize that it may mean that you are not eating a balanced diet and spend a few days eating really healthily; you will probably find the cravings disappear all by themselves (*see* chapter 8 on healthy eating guidelines).
  - Finally, if you really want something sweet to eat, such as chocolate, aim to have it after a meal which is high in complex carbohydrates, rather than eating it on an empty stomach. If you do this, your blood sugar level will be maintained by the complex carbohydrates and the chocolate will not stimulate overproduction of insulin, which will result in subsequent feelings of hunger and associated cravings for more chocolate.

- **Have a variety of food tastes.** In traditional Indian medicine, it is believed that there are six different tastes – sweet, sour, salty, bitter, pungent and astringent – and that if your diet contains all of these you will have a balanced, natural diet. Even if you do not agree with this completely, it can be useful to have a range of food tastes in your meals to keep your taste buds stimulated and your stomach satisfied.

- **Recognize thirst as well as hunger.** Often, when we think we need food, what we really need is water. Your mind may not be good at distinguishing between the two needs, so each time you think you need to eat, just check – maybe all you need is a refreshing drink of water. It can be useful to check this before each meal; it *may* take the edge off your appetite and stop you overeating if you drink a glass of water a quarter of an hour or so before a meal. However, if you are really hungry you should actually be eating, not just drinking water now in order to eat more later.

- **Allow your body time to give you information.** As I said earlier, it may take around 20 minutes after you eat before your brain receives the message that your stomach is full. So do allow time for your food to begin being digested and only eat more if after half an hour or so you still really feel hungry.

In this chapter I have given you ways of using your own motivational patterns in your weight-control programme. The next chapter will help get you started.

6
Putting Your Plans Into Action

> *This chapter is about how you can put what you have learned in this book into operation. I will be giving you some practical techniques for planning and organizing, finding role models, getting information, taking action and monitoring your progress.*

So far, we have talked about motivation and about various techniques which you can use to make changes. To be successful, however, you need to have ways of making a start, keeping on track and assessing how far you have got. This chapter will give you some ideas on doing just that.

Making a start: setting goals

Setting your goals is an essential first step. As we discussed earlier, it is important to have goals which will work for you. The previous chapter gave you ideas on setting goals which are in keeping with your own motivational patterns, so do follow the advice and make your goals as clear, precise and measurable as you can.

Planning and organizing

Planning is a vital part of the process of weight control. If you do not plan, it is easier to be diverted. For example, if you are travelling, it is easy to fall for high-fat fast food unless you have taken some healthier things with you to eat. If you do not plan, it is easier to eat junk food at home because you do not have any fresh food in the house. If you do not plan, it is easier to snack while shopping if you have gone out on an empty stomach.

If you do plan, however, it is easier to:

- list all the foods to buy, so you make sure to get the healthier options
- eat before shopping, so that you are not going out on an empty stomach and being tempted to nibble as you go along
- keep a fridge full of healthy snacks for those times when you feel you just must have something
- prepare menus in advance so that they are balanced and contain a good selection of items
- organize yourself to exercise at regular times
- think ahead to events so that you can decide in advance how to cope with them

There are lots of aids to planning and I will tell you about some simple ones now.

Charts

A good way to plan is to have a chart on the wall, on which you can enter the things you intend to do. You can buy wall planners from stationery shops, you can use a calendar or you can make up something to your own design. Make sure your chart has a space for each day, with room to write in.

When you have your chart, you can use it to put in a whole variety of things – for example, the days and times when you will exercise, the things you need to buy at the shops, the people you need to telephone to tell them how well you are doing. You can make your charts very personal, with pictures, coloured writing, cuttings and so on – whatever works for you is best.

The advantage of charts is that they are easy to see at a glance.

Diaries

As an alternative to a chart, you can make notes in a diary of what you intend to do.

The advantage is that it is easy to carry with you and refer to quickly.

Computers

You could keep a note of things to do on your computer, which can be fun if you enjoy playing with equipment.

The advantage of computers is that they are easy to update and you can print copies of your plan.

Lists

You can keep lists of what to do, and check things off as you do them. Your list might be in a notebook, pinned up on the wall, stuck to the fridge with a magnet or whatever other method you find best.

The advantage of a list is that it gives you the detail you need to be well organized.

If you are not a person who finds planning easy, you might like to enlist the help of a friend who can help you with the process. Maybe you could trade off something which you could do in return.

Organizing your time, your environment and the resources around you

Getting yourself really well organized is the key to successful management of weight. I have already told you about aids to planning; here are some things you can use to help you get some order into the way you approach things.

- Get support from others living with you; make sure they understand what you are aiming for and agree to help. This may mean making arrangements to eat together so that you are not cooking several meals every day, each with opportunities for you to nibble.
- Sort out your kitchen cupboards and remove any tempting foods which should not be there.
- Plan food-shopping trips at times when you have just eaten and will not be tempted to snack.
- Keep all the foods you need in stock so that you can prepare really balanced, nutritious meals.

Finding a role model

A good way to be successful is to find other people who are successful already and copy some of what they do. This is not about becoming another person, but simply adopting some of that person's behaviour.

What are some of the things you might copy? At the beginning of the book, I said that results come from a combination of factors, including having well-specified goals, having the behavioural skills which are necessary, and having positive and supportive thoughts, feelings and beliefs. So when you find your role models, you can copy what they do in any of these areas.

141

For example, you might find out exactly how they set themselves goals. Do they work to short- or long-term time scales? Do they keep renewing their goals so that as one is achieved another is substituted? Do they have goals for having fun as well as for working hard?

Regarding behaviour, you might find out whether they eat certain kinds of food, whether they shop at a certain time of day or whether they have a particular thing they do when they feel a food craving coming on. And as far as thoughts, feelings and beliefs go, you could find out what goes through their minds as they think about managing their diet and exercise, how they feel when they are successful and what they believe about how they will be in the future.

By having more than one role model, you can find a range of successful behaviour patterns and see what common threads run through them. You can also select those behaviours which seem to fit best with your own lifestyle.

By the way, your role models do not need to be people you know personally; they may be people you have seen on TV or have read about in books. Do remember, though, that if your role models are not people you can actually speak to, you may only be able to find out about some aspects of what they do, so finding 'live' role models is likely to be more productive.

Getting information

Before you embark on your programme, there may well be some information you need. Some of the things which will be helpful are as follows:

- advice from your doctor if you have not embarked on a fitness programme recently or if you are very overweight or have any health problems which might be affected by changes in diet or exercise
- details of a local fitness centre
- stockists of specialist foods
- product information on items you would like to purchase for your programme

Taking action

Take one step at a time. You can complete even the largest task if you break it down into suitably sized chunks. Work towards daily or weekly goals rather than only the long-term ones. Take each day as it comes and be pleased that you have achieved even small successes within each day. You can imagine even the biggest sea as being made up of single drops of water. Every drop counts – and it is the same with your programme.

And as you take action, really *be aware* of what you are doing. This will make it real and ensure that you will not be sidetracked.

Monitoring your progress

It is important to check how you are doing as you go along. There are various reasons for this: it will keep you motivated, it will show you whether there are changes in your speed of progress and, as you achieve your original goals, it will allow you to decide if you need to set new objectives for the future.

To help you assess your progress you can do the following:

- **Set yourself review dates.** Weekly reviews are probably the most effective; they give you adequate time to make progress and are a constant reminder of how you are doing.
- **Work out suitable assessment processes.** Sometimes people feel they have to keep weighing themselves in order to check on their progress. Frequent weighing can be misleading, because water retention may vary from day to day, showing weight fluctuations and, as you lose fat and develop more muscle, you can weigh more but actually be better toned and fitter. So constant weighing can give you misleading results. You may prefer to forget weighing altogether and rely on looking at yourself in the mirror, or checking whether your clothes are becoming looser on you. These checks are probably more useful and will also get you into the habit of really seeing the progress you make.
- **Make sure you take notice of results.** For example, look at your charts and in the mirror to see your progress. Listen to what others are saying about how well you are doing and notice how much better you feel as you make progress.

To help you monitor your success, make yourself an action plan. It is good to have four columns on the plan, which can take up one sheet of paper. Make the first column a space to list all the things you intend to do. The second column is for you to put a time scale in for each action you intend to take. The third column is to list any resources you need, such as the support of friends or family. The last column is to enter the results you expect – in other words how you would like things to be when you have reached each goal. By keeping your plan up-dated on a regular basis, you will be able to keep on track and see how well you are doing from week to week.

GOAL	TIME SCALE	RESOURCES	RESULTS
Walk for 20 mins.	Each Friday	Good shoes	2 months later, gone each week
Eat more vegetables	Daily	Adequate shopping time	Eating at least 2 vegetables daily

In this chapter I have given you ways of starting and maintaining your programme. Once you begin, you will find it becomes easier and, the more results you get, the more you will be motivated to continue achieving. But what about those times when it is not so easy to keep going? The next chapter will give you some ideas on how to keep on track in less easy times.

7

Keeping on Track

> We all have times when we become diverted from our goals; this chapter will give you ways of keeping on track and overcoming obstacles which may appear to stand in your way.

Sometimes things may prevent you from achieving what you set out to do. You will have your own ideas on this and if you think about these things in advance it is easier to overcome them. And, by the way, if you think of space flights, it is interesting to know that they are actually slightly off course for much of the time; the art in getting them to their destination is making constant tiny adjustments to keep them on track.

So what could divert you from your goals?

Well-meaning advice from friends

Most of us have friends who try to give us help in what we do. Usually it is well intended although, on occasion, if you are doing really well, someone might be tempted to suggest things which could actually throw you off track because they are jealous of what you are achieving.

Well-meaning advice can come in many forms. Do any of these sound familiar?

- 'Oh, just have one; it won't do you any harm.'
- 'What I found really useful was ...'
- 'You really ought to have a go at ...'

- 'You don't want to overdo exercise; you might strain something.'
- 'It doesn't matter if you weigh . . . ; I weigh . . . and I'm OK.'
- 'You might get really tired if you don't eat more than that.'
- 'Chocolate is really good for you; it gives you energy.'
- 'I heard on the television that eating 2lb/1kg of . . . every day makes you lose weight faster.'
- 'The only way to lose weight is to take pills that stop you feeling hungry.'
- 'If you really want to improve something, why not go to an evening class and learn a new language, rather than doing aerobics?'

Many such comments are well meant, but can put you off what you are doing or divert you into activities which may not be beneficial.

If your friends give you unsuitable advice, it helps to have some answers ready. Some you might find helpful are:

- 'Even one will make a difference; every bit counts when you're working to a plan.'
- 'I know that really helped *you*, but I'm different, and what works for *me* is . . .'
- 'That sounds interesting, but I'm happy with what I'm doing right now.'
- 'I've got really good at knowing how much I can do; I stop if I feel I'm likely to overdo things.'
- 'I'm glad you're happy with your weight; I would prefer to be . . .'
- 'Actually, eating the right foods gives me more energy rather than less.'

147

- 'You can't believe all you hear on TV; it may work, but I don't think anyone has found a single miracle food yet.'
- 'Pills may work for some people, but I prefer to eat fresh foods that will keep me healthy long term, rather than going for a quick fix that could wear off shortly.'
- 'Because what I have decided to do at this stage is to improve my body; when I've done that I can improve my language skills.'

How many other answers can you think of to these comments, and how many other things can you predict that people will say to 'help' you? Knowing in your own mind how to answer means that you have thought clearly about what you want to achieve and are convinced that you will get there. Once that has happened, it is easy to convince others that you mean business.

Special events with tempting foods

We all know about these: the meal out at a special restaurant, the birthday lunch, the engagement party, the retirement do and so on. All of them seem to be accompanied by food – and often high-fat, processed food – and high-calorie alcoholic drinks.

When you are keeping to your weight-control plan, you can still go to these events, but it helps to have thought out what to do to keep to your plan. Some things you can do include:

- eating something beforehand so you will not feel so tempted to indulge in things which are not on your list of acceptable foods

- eating what everyone else eats, but only having very small portions
- selecting only the low-fat parts of the meal; this is usually possible unless absolutely everything is high in fat
- eating very slowly, so people are not tempted to put more on your plate
- avoiding alcoholic drinks and keeping to mineral water (fruit juice is good in small quantities, but be careful about overdoing it, as most fruit juice is high in calories)
- telling people (in advance if possible) that you are on a weight-control programme and that you will only be eating certain foods, or small amounts
- drinking a lot of water before eating, so you feel full and do not want so much to eat
- if it is a buffet meat, getting there a bit later, so most people have already eaten and it will not be so notice-able if you avoid eating too much

How many other options can you think of for dealing with these events?

Lapses

It is only human to lapse from time to time; we are not machines and do not always do things in the same way. It is your attitude to lapses which is most important. A single lapse will not affect your programme much; better to face the fact that you have done whatever it is and decide to keep to your programme from then on.

Keeping a note of lapses, and finding out how and when they occur, will help you in the future. If you find you are more likely to succumb to snacks late at night, plan to keep some healthy options in the fridge so you can have them instead. If you find you are tempted by cake and sweets in the supermarket, get a friend to come with you and put you off buying them! By anticipating lapses and planning to deal with them, you will become more resourceful and better able to cope.

Low self-esteem and negative beliefs

I talked about motivation in chapter 3 and discussed some of the factors which influence it. If you believe you have value as a person and deserve to succeed, it is easier to get on. Occasionally, however, you may start to feel you are not worth an investment of time and effort.

To get over this, you might like to have a go at these activities.

Using affirmations

Affirmations involve repeating positive things to yourself on a regular basis, for example: 'I am making real progress'; 'I am in control of my programme'; 'I am a capable person'; 'I deserve to succeed'. Affirmations work best when you put them in the present tense; that means saying '*I am*' rather than '*I will*'. When you repeat them several times every day the message goes through to your mind that what you are saying is true. And when you really believe you are worthy of effort and capable of success, results will come more quickly. You will already have come across some affirmations in chapter 5 where we covered ways of changing limiting beliefs into more positive ones.

Recognizing past results

Another thing which can help is for you to recognize that you have already been successful at other things in the past. So take a sheet of paper and jot down as many things as possible that you can remember doing well. These might be things you did at school, with your family, in hobbies or pastimes, or at work. You might like to extend this a little and, against each thing, write down the skill or ability which enabled you to do it. For example, you might put: 'I taught my child to do up his shoelaces, which needed patience and cheerfulness as well as clear explanations and demonstration.' This might sound a small example, but the more you think, the more examples you will find of times when you did things really well in the past. You may also find out about some abilities you did not realize you had.

Noting present results

Now you can think of things you continue to be successful at. They do not need to be major things; even small ones can give you a real sense of achievement. A good way of recognizing this is to start with an exercise like the following.

Get a large envelope and some small pieces of paper. Every day for a week, find five or six things that you are doing well. For example you might have made a really good cup of tea, you might have cheered a friend up on the phone and you might have avoided running over a cat by braking quickly in your car. Each time you notice yourself doing something well, write it down on a piece of paper and put it in the envelope. At the end of the week, open the envelope and notice all the things you have done really well that week. A simple exercise like

151

this can really make you aware of just how successful you can be and, once you know you can do small things successfully, you will know you have the ability to do bigger things well too.

Using visual reminders or sounds

This is a good way of helping yourself to keep on track. Visual reminders can include photographs which you can pin on the wall, posters, 'post-it' notes with messages on (for example on your fridge, or on the doors of your wardrobe). You can also have 'success barometers', which show you your progress to date; these might be charts or they might have pictures such as an outline of a person which you can make smaller as you lose weight.

If you do not like the idea of visual reminders, you can substitute ones with sounds. For example in a recent mail-order catalogue one product was a plastic cockerel with a battery in, which crowed every time it sensed a movement. You might like to have something like that which gives you a cheerful sound to keep you motivated.

Support and encouragement

Having support for what they do is very important to many people. If you build a network of friends and family who can help you in your efforts, it can be very useful. You may have a special friend you can telephone when you need a little encouragement. You may have a pen-pal or Internet contact you can correspond with. You may have a partner who you can talk to and tell about your difficulties and your achievements.

And, if you do not already have people you can get this support from, there are other options, such as weight-control classes, leisure centres with helpful instructors and advice lines. And if you feel you need real support in times of what seems like crisis, many countries have telephone lines which members of the public can ring for general advice, support and counselling.

Animal days

We all have days when things just do not seem to go right. It can help to think of such days in an amusing way, rather than getting upset about them. One way of doing this is to think about 'animal days'.

Each species of animal has its own individual characteristics, which includes their responses to food and their responses to activity. Various kinds of animal are listed below, each with its own typical approach to food and exercise. Now, while these approaches are entirely suitable for the animals in question, they are not so appropriate for people! So have a look at them and see if any of them sound like you on a bad day! You might also like to add your own animal types to the list. Next time you have a small lapse in your programme, just think of it as an 'animal day' – perhaps a 'goldfish day' or a 'butterfly day' – and plan to do things differently tomorrow.

Animal food days

- **Goldfish.** Goldfish are active and much of their life is taken up with a search for food. Goldfish seem to be greedy and eat all the time.
- **Snake.** Snakes use little energy and are very good at making the most of their food supplies. Snakes eat very infrequently; sometimes apparently too little to sustain them.

- **Cat.** Cats are extremely selective about their food; it has to be just the right kind, just the right temperature and offered at just the right time. Cats can be fussy or faddy about their food.
- **Dog.** Dogs are somewhat undiscriminating about their food; if it will go in their mouth they are likely to eat it, even if it seems revolting to us and the kind of thing which really should not be going into any stomach.
- **Goat.** Goats utilize whatever they can lay their eyes on; they will eat practically anything, even if it is the first thing they see.
- **Panda.** Pandas have a very limited diet; it is said they only eat bamboo, which can seem unbalanced on the face of it.
- **Bird.** Birds need to create enormous amounts of energy to cope with flying and looking after their youngsters; they eat tiny amounts and are constantly 'picking'.
- **Squirrel.** Squirrels have to put food by in the good weather so they can get through colder spells; they hoard food 'just in case' times are hard.

Animal exercise days

- **Snail.** Snails move very slowly; it takes them ages to get anywhere.
- **Bluebottle.** Bluebottles buzz around a lot, often going around in circles and not really getting anywhere.
- **Elephant.** Elephants are heavy animals and have to put a lot of effort into moving.
- **Butterfly.** Butterflies flit from one thing to another, never settling on anything for very long.

- **Hamster.** Hamsters go round and round on treadmills, thinking they are going somewhere but actually not seeing beyond the wheel in front of them.
- **Rabbit.** Rabbits are on the hop all the time, always on the go.

Of course animals do not spend all their time in activities which do not get anywhere, but thinking about things in a more lighthearted way like this sometimes really helps to get them in perspective.

Looking good

While you are slimming, you will probably find it gives you a boost if you know you look good. Making the most of yourself is possible whatever your weight and, if you know a few of the 'tricks of the trade', you can give your ego a real boost. Here are some of the things you can do:

- **Wear colours which flatter you.** When you wear the right colours, you will find you look better. Colours which flatter you make you look more energetic, give your skin a nice tone and balance your appearance. Choose colours which complement your own colouring; if you are very dark, choose deep colours, and if you are lighter in colouring, choose lighter colours. If your hair is black, dark brown, mousy or ash blonde, choose colours with a blue base and if your hair is red, golden brown, auburn or honey blonde choose colours with a yellow base.
- **Wear shapes which flatter you.** Shapes which are flattering complement your proportions. So, if you are large boned, choose big, bold shapes; if small boned, choose smaller, neater shapes. If you have a

155

round face, wear necklines which are soft, but a little cut away so that you do not exaggerate the roundness; if you have a long face, avoid necklines which are very deeply V-shaped, as they will exaggerate the length.

- **Wear make-up and accessories which complement your clothes and your natural colouring.** This means wearing gold if you have a warm colouring and silver if you have a cool colouring. It means wearing small, neat accessories if you are small and small boned and larger accessories if you are bigger. It means having shoes and bags in tones which complement your clothes, rather than vying with them.
- **Wear clothes which fit well.** If you are large, avoid clothes which are tight; they will crease and look untidy and are likely to accentuate fat rather than hide it. Go for clothes which are well cut and hang nicely rather than cling.
- **Make the most of focal points and optical illusions.** Rather than hide yourself under acres of black in the hope that it will disguise your extra weight, place well-chosen items at strategic points to draw attention away from problem areas. For example, if your hips are large, wear a colourful scarf or some attractive earrings – people will notice them rather than looking at your hips. And if you are short, either wear clothes all of the same colour (ie blouse, skirt, shoes) or wear brighter, lighter colours above your waist and darker ones below to draw other people's eyes upwards, thus making you appear taller.

There are many other tips of this kind and in the Bibliography you will find details of tapes which will give you more information on how to look good, whatever your size.

And finally, two important things to remember ...

Plateaux

Many people find they reach a stage in their weight-control programme where they do not seem to be making progress any more. This is often referred to as a 'plateau', and what happens is that weight reduction either decreases or stops. But it is important to remember that this is only a *temporary* stage, and it *will* pass.

Plateaux occur because your body physiology is re-adjusting itself and taking time to accustom itself to a new eating pattern. And you can be especially likely to reach a plateau if you cut calories without taking adequate exercise; this can lead you to burn calories more slowly and take longer to achieve results.

In some ways, it is like what happens to some marathon runners, which they refer to as 'hitting the wall'. The physiological reasons for this temporary feeling of being unable to continue are not the same as with weight loss, but the effect can be similar – a feeling of being demotivated and unable to continue. By persevering and maintaining your good eating and exercise habits, you will soon begin to lose weight again and be really pleased you decided to carry on.

Giving yourself rewards

Rewards can be excellent for keeping you on track. You can have fun choosing the kind of reward you would like and deciding when you will present it to yourself. Things that some people have used include a visit to a special place, a massage, a new outfit, an audiotape or CD, a picture for the wall or a plant for the garden.

You might break down your rewards into sections. For example one thing which can work well is to have a favourite book which you read while on an exercise bike. By only allowing yourself to read the book while you are exercising, you can motivate yourself to continue.

And finally, the best reward is to bring one hand over the opposite shoulder and give yourself a big pat on the back.

This chapter has given you ways of keeping to your plans. The more you want to achieve results the more likely it is that you will do so, and the better you plan for success the more likely it is you will achieve it.

There is just one thing left now, and that is information about healthy living. Whatever programme you choose to follow, it will help if you have some guidelines about healthy eating and beneficial exercise. In the final chapter, I take you through currently accepted ideas about these topics.

8
Diet, Exercise and Therapies

| *This chapter gives you information and guidance on food and lifestyle.*

Diet

Food gives us the building blocks of life. It gives us energy and the essential nutrients we need to keep our bodies going.

I use the word 'diet' here as a description of what you eat and not to mean a restricted programme of calorie counted meals. Calorie counting has been shown not to be a very effective way of losing weight, because emphasis is put solely on calorie levels and not on educating you to a healthy way of life. This book is not about measuring the food you eat in exact detail; it is about encouraging you to move to a balance in your diet and in the exercise you take. When you do this you will find your weight is controlled naturally and you won't need to spend time noting the calorie content of every morsel you put in your mouth.

Healthy eating
Human beings are designed to utilize a wide range of foods. Unlike certain animals, which can exist on only a very limited range of nutrients, people are able to eat

and benefit from many different things. For example, we can be vegetarian or eat meat; we can eat food hot, warm or cold; we can eat sweet things or savoury things; we can eat natural foods or processed foods.

Unfortunately, the ability to be flexible with your diet means that you may well eat things which are not particularly good for you, simply because they are readily available, or because you have developed a taste for them. Healthy eating is about eating foods which do our bodies good, not harm.

In his book, *Reversing Ageing*, Dr Paul Galbraith says that eating unhealthily results in premature ageing, chronic fatigue, degenerative diseases, reduced immunity to disease and obesity. So what we eat can have major effects on our lives.

A balanced diet

While you could exist on a limited range of nutrients, you would probably be missing some things which contribute to good body function. In order to be really healthy, it is important to balance your diet; in other words to take in a combination of all the different food elements which you require to enable your body to work well. The major elements of food you need are:

- carbohydrates
- protein
- fats
- vitamins
- minerals

Fibre and water are also essential elements of a healthy diet (*see* later in this chapter for more on these) and it is generally held that a wholefood diet, where all the essential elements are contained in a manner as close as possible to their natural state, is best.

Let us take each of the food elements and see where they can be found.

Carbohydrates

Carbohydrates are found in foods such as bread, pasta, rice and other grains, potatoes, fruits and vegetables, and products with sugar in. There are simple carbohydrates, such as sugar, which are quickly absorbed by the body, and complex carbohydrates, such as potatoes, pasta and grains, which generally take longer to work through your system. The simple carbohydrates often lead to feelings of hunger soon after eating, because the carbohydrates turn into sugars quickly, leading to immediate feelings of energy and wellbeing, but also subsequent hunger and tiredness. The complex carbohydrates, in contrast, usually break down more slowly in your body and so keep you feeling well nourished for longer (*see* Appendix).

Diet books always used to tell people to cut down on carbohydrates if they wanted to lose weight, but actually complex carbohydrates are good in a weight-control programme as they stave off hunger for long periods, helping you resist the temptation to eat more than you need. Carbohydrates contain both starch and fibre and fibre helps prevent constipation and reduces the risk of some common disorders of the intestine. In addition, certain carbohydrates (oats, beans, lentils, fruit and vegetables) may also help to reduce the amount of harmful cholesterol in your blood. It is now generally held that starchy foods should make up at least half of your diet.

Apart from this being a guideline for healthy eating,

there is another reason why carbohydrates are good for us. There is a newish science with a rather long name; psychoneuroimmunology (sometimes referred to as PNI for short). According to this, there are very close links between how our minds function and how healthy we are; when we are positive and feel good, our immune system (the body's defence against illness) is much stronger. There is evidence that some foods (and some carbohydrates in particular) have a strong effect on our mental approach, making us feel good, so a diet high in carbohydrates can strengthen our resistance to illness as well as helping us lose weight.

Protein
Protein is found in fish, meat, poultry and meat, and in dairy products such as milk, cheese and eggs. It is also found in some vegetable sources, including nuts and seeds, grains, beans, and vegetable products such as soya and sprouted seeds. It used to be thought that high amounts of protein were necessary, and that a high-protein diet helped you to lose weight faster. Nowadays it is generally believed that a high-protein diet is not needed for good health; smaller amounts of protein are adequate, and around a tenth of your total diet is probably adequate for protein intake.

Fats
There are three main kinds of fat.

- saturated fats (found in meat and in dairy products, such as lard, milk, butter, cream and cheese and also in cakes and biscuits, pies and chips), which tend to be solid at room temperature

- monounsaturated fats (found in fish oils, peanuts, olive and vegetable oils)
- polyunsaturated fats (found in vegetables, soya, sunflower, corn and sesame seeds, as well as in some margarines and in oily fish such as sardines, mackerel and salmon); these do have many benefits and some in particular have been shown to have an important part to play in protecting against heart disease.

There are other fats too, but these are the main ones you need to know about.

Although fats are essential to a balanced diet, too much fat is a major cause of excess weight. Fat contains proportionately more calories than the same weight of other kinds of food, so eating a small amount of butter or cheese will give far more calories than the same weight of fruit, vegetables or fish. In addition, saturated fats can produce high levels of certain cholesterol, which can build up in the arteries. There are links between high consumption of these fats and heart problems and cancers. Monounsaturated fats, such as those found in olive oil, are thought to be healthier and polyunsaturated fats may actually help to change the ratio of cholesterol levels in the body for the better – increasing HDL ('good' cholesterol) can actually a benefit to health.

In general, it is felt that fats should make up no more than a third of your diet.

Vitamins and minerals

Vitamins and minerals are found in a wide range of foods and they are essential to healthy life. If your diet is deficient in vitamins and minerals you will soon succumb to illness. The best source of vitamins is fresh food, although you may feel you need to take a manufactured food supplement (*see* page 17).

The value of vitamins and minerals can be affected by many things. If food is prepared too early, its vitamin content diminishes rapidly as cut surfaces are exposed to air, light and heat; overcooking also reduces vitamin and mineral value. Boiling, especially, can have the effect of leaching vitamins and water-soluble minerals into the surrounding water, so steaming or – especially with fruit and vegetables – eating food raw is much better nutritionally. Storage also has an effect, because keeping food for lengthy periods can reduce its vitamin and mineral levels. Keeping food hot for a long time also reduces vitamin levels.

Another way in which you can make the most of the vitamin and mineral content of foods is by juicing fruit and vegetables. Having a food juicer is an excellent way of making sure you have a daily supply of essential nutrients, and there are some wonderful combinations of foods which you can have in this way. You should take time to get used to fruit and vegetable juices, however, by starting with small amounts only.

Another important thing to know about vitamins and minerals is that their effectiveness can sometimes be reduced unless they are combined correctly. For example, calcium, which is an important factor in bone growth, needs the presence of certain other elements, including vitamin D, if it is to be absorbed well by the body. Drinking tea with a meal can inhibit iron absorbtion and there are many other particular combinations of foods which either enhance or reduce the body's ability to absorb and utilize essential vitamins and minerals. If you are interested in knowing more about this, there are many specialist publications on nutrition currently available.

Therefore, a healthy diet includes all the main categories of food and, when you balance all these well, you are more likely to have a healthy life and avoid illness. So what are the best sources of each of the food elements? They include fruit, vegetables, meat, fish, poultry, dairy products, bread, grains, pulses and vegetable products. Let's look at each of these in turn.

Fruit and vegetables

Fruit and vegetables are excellent for maintaining health. Although all food elements are essential to a balanced diet, there is no doubt that eating plenty of fruit and vegetables is one of the best things you can do to keep fit and healthy as they are packed with vital nutrients. Moreover, because, with very few exceptions, most fruit and vegetables do not contain fat, a diet high in these foodstuffs makes a major contribution to any weight loss programme. I suggest you eat a minimum of five portions of fresh fruit and vegetables each day, where a portion could be half a grapefruit, an apple, a banana, a glass of fruit juice, 3–4oz/100g of vegetables or a small bowl of salad.

It is also useful to remember that many fruits, such as grapes or dried fruits, contain high levels of natural sugars (and, therefore, calories), so it is best to have both fruit and vegetables in your diet, rather than fruit only.

In addition to their usefulness in a weight-control programme, fruit and vegetables help protect your body against illness and increase its defence mechanisms. The way they do this is by providing you with what are known as antioxidants. Antioxidants prevent oils, fats and fat-soluble vitamins in food from combining with oxygen and becoming rancid. It is now generally accepted that elements called free radicals exist in our environment. Free radicals have been described as highly reactive types of oxygen, resulting from air pollution, excessive exposure to sun, tobacco, barbecued meat, red wine and other processes. When active in our bodies, they combine with oxygen to oxidize various compounds, producing a detrimental effect on long-term health. It is believed that oxidization is a major contributory factor to such things as premature ageing and the development of cancer, so that anything which can reduce this effect will be beneficial.

Antioxidants counter this process and eating foods high in antioxidants is one way of preventing harmful oxidization in our bodies. The foods which are high in antioxidants include fresh fruit and vegetables. Eating a high proportion of these foods, and especially eating them raw, is said to have a major effect on enhancing the body's immune system and fighting free radicals.

To maintain high levels of antioxidants in your body, it is recommended that your diet includes highly coloured foods, such as bright-green leafy vegetables (eg broccoli, sprouts and dark cabbage) and orange/red/yellow vegetables (eg carrot, beetroot and tomato).

Vegetable products

There is an increasing variety of vegetable products on the market now and many of these are very helpful in maintaining a healthy diet. Examples include tofu and soya (soya milk, soya curd and soya flour), from which are made many different products. These products are especially useful for vegetarians and vegans, who find they are a valuable addition to their diets as well as providing the base for a wide range of menus. All these products are low fat and therefore contain far fewer calories than traditional meat- , fish- or poultry-based meals.

Dairy products

Dairy products are generally recommended as part of a balanced diet, especially because of their contribution as an excellent source of calcium, which is vital for bone growth, especially in children. However, calcium may not be absorbed easily from dairy products, and some people consider that they should not be consumed by adults as they may cause excess mucus formation, which can lead to breathing problems.

Some dairy products have very high fat contents (full-fat milk, cream and cream cheese) and it is useful to know that lower-fat dairy products still have the same (or sometimes higher) amounts of calcium. So, for example, you can obtain similar amounts of calcium from ½pt/300ml of full-fat milk, ½pt/300ml of skimmed milk or a small tub of yoghurt. (Although it is important to know, however, that certain foods can contribute towards calcium being leached out of the body. For example fibre tends to bind calcium, making it inaccessible for use by the body.) It is worth checking on this if you want to protect your bones from the disabling problem of osteoporosis.

Meat and meat products

Opinion is also divided about the nutritional value of meat and meat products, although meat is an excellent source of protein. It is generally recommended that your diet should not contain excessive amounts of red meat and that white meat is better. And, as a good deal of fat is found just under the skin on many animals, it is recommended that, for a low-fat diet, any skin and fat should be cut off before cooking.

Meat products are very varied nutritionally. Many, such as bacon, sausages and salamis are very high in fat (and also in salt), and are not a great help in weight control because they are high in calories and could also encourage water retention because of their high salt content. If you are going to eat meat, it is best to have it unprocessed, so that you gain the maximum benefits from the elements it does contain.

Poultry

Poultry is generally considered good in a diet, although you have to be careful about its source. Factory-farmed birds (as with other farm animals) may be given drugs, such as antibiotics, which can be absorbed by our bodies if they are still in the animal's system when we eat it. It is best to go for free-range, organically farmed animals wherever possible; they usually taste better and are less likely to have harmful drugs inside them.

Turkey is an excellent source of low-fat meat but, again, be careful to avoid the oversized, factory-reared birds, which often suffer physical defects resulting from the way in which they are kept. Organically farmed animals may be more expensive, but are better for us and are reared more humanely.

As with meat, you should ensure that you cut off the skin of poultry before cooking, so as to remove the fat just under it.

Grains, grain products, nuts and seeds

There are many kinds of grains (including wheat, rye, barley, oats, rice), seeds (eg pumpkin, sunflower and sesame) and nuts (eg walnuts and hazelnuts) and many nutritious products such as bread and pasta can be made from them. Grains, nuts and seeds provide protein, fibre, vitamins and minerals and are an essential foundation for a healthy diet, although nuts can have a very high oil content and should be used sparingly in a weight-control programme. Grains are often highly processed, which often removes much of their nutritional value and benefit, but in a natural state wholegrains are extremely nutritious.

Pulses

Pulses are another important element of a balanced diet. They include fresh beans and peas and also dried ones, such as lentils, chickpeas, butter beans and kidney beans. Most dried pulses need soaking for a few hours before cooking.

Water

Water is a basic foundation for life. Around 70 per cent of our bodies is made up of water, without which we would become dehydrated and die. Actually, water is a basic ingredient for life as a whole and it is the fact that the earth has such a plentiful supply of water that enables it to sustain life as we know it.

Water can be obtained by the body in three ways. We can get it through drinking, through eating foods with a water content and by absorbing tiny amounts into the skin. In fact if you do not drink reasonable quantities of water on a regular basis your skin is likely to become dehydrated and look in poor condition.

Many foods have a high water content, including fruits and vegetables which, eaten raw or lightly cooked, provide us with a high proportion of our daily fluid intake. Overcooking, especially in an oven, can lead to food becoming dried out and of less value as far as its water content is concerned.

The best way of taking in water, however, is to drink it. It is important that it is pure water; drinks such as tea and coffee, although high in water, are also high in caffeine and caffeine can act as a diuretic, which means that you excrete a high proportion of the water you have drunk and possibly more besides.

The amount of water you need to drink will vary, depending on factors such as climate, the energy you expend and the amount of high-water-content food you eat. On the whole, most sources recommend a daily intake of at least 2 pints/1 litre of water and up to 3½ pints/2 litres or more, especially in dry weather, if your body is to have the hydration it needs. And remember that, odd though it sounds, if you wait until you feel thirsty before drinking water, your body is already dehydrated to some extent; so make sure you keep up your fluid intake unless there is a medical reason for you to do otherwise.

Food supplements

Medical opinion is still divided between those who believe that a balanced diet does not need any kind of supplementation and those who believe that, however healthily we may try to eat, our food may be low in nutrients. This can be either because it is grown on poor soil with overuse of chemicals, or because storage and transportation times, combined with processing and cooking, may deplete the food's essential nutrients. In such cases, it is argued, it is necessary to take supplements to replace these deficiencies.

If you are wondering whether you need to supplement your diet in some way, you might like to ask yourself the following questions:

- Do I lack energy and get tired easily?
- Are my skin, hair and nails in poor condition?
- Do I easily catch colds, flu and other ailments?
- Do I have frequent mood swings, bouts of depression or irritability?

If you have answered 'Yes' to any of these questions, it may be that you need to look at your diet to see if you are getting all the nourishment you need. If you *are* eating a balanced diet, with sufficient amounts of each of the elements I mentioned above, you may need some supplementation. You may also benefit from some increased exercise, and I will be turning to this shortly. It is also possible that you could benefit from supplements if your bone density is decreasing (osteoporosis); you would need medical advice, however, on whether this was the case and, if so, what supplements – or other remedial actions – were recommended.

What supplements are available?

If you do decide to add supplements to your diet, there is an almost overwhelming variety and range to choose from. There are natural supplements, ones which are artificial in their origin, and pills, drinks and complete foods designed to augment other parts of your diet.

It is important that you take advice on supplementation before adding to your diet in this way, and there are various sources of help. Some of the things you might do include:

- asking your doctor what he or she would recommend
- asking your pharmacist for advice
- finding a nutritionist who can give you advice
- calling a specialist health advice line (*see* Useful Addresses for information on this)
- reading a specialist book on food supplementation

You may find that the advice from these sources can be very variable so, after taking advice, you will probably still have to decide for yourself what the most appropriate course of action will be.

How much should you eat?

It is difficult to generalize about this, as people's metabolic rates (the rate at which they burn up food and turn it into energy) vary so much. In addition, some people have different levels of activity and therefore need a higher food intake. Very young people will need a higher intake to fuel their growth levels (including especially for babies and very young children, a proportionally higher fat intake than would be suitable for adults).

You may have come across guidelines on calorie intake which are generally based on whether you are a man or a woman, large or small boned, and more or less active. However, as I said earlier, calorie counting is *not* the way to manage your weight. What you need to do is to listen to what your body says it needs, eat when you are hungry and not when you are not and have a good balance of nutrients to give you sustained energy – and using your mind positively will help you achieve this.

To check when you need to eat, it is good to take a few moments before eating to consider whether you really are hungry, or just want food because it is there, because of habit or because it is a substitute for something else. Taking time to do this so that you only eat when you really *are* hungry is the best thing you can do to help your programme go well.

An interesting fact is that some research studies have shown that animals accustomed to very low amounts of food tend to live longer. This is not an argument for the very low-calorie diets which I mentioned in chapter 1, but for avoiding overconsumption, which makes your body sluggish and your mind less active.

Another interesting fact is that we in the West seem to be eating *less* than we used to overall, despite the common weight gains found in a high percentage of the population. Apparently we eat between a quarter and a third fewer calories nowadays than we did 30 years ago, but we are still getting heavier. There are different explanations for this, one being that people nowadays take less exercise than they used to (for example, household chores now are often mechanized, with washing machines, food mixers, gas fires etc) and jobs are often desk-bound rather than manual. But a particular explanation for the increases in weight is that they are related to the *type* rather than the quantity of food eaten. We eat much more fat than we used to (double the quantity in the British diet over the past 50 years according to the Dunn Clinical Nutrition Institute). Because fat does not make us feel as full as carbohydrates, we eat more of it in order to feel full.

When should you eat

There are some differing views about when to eat, but the general view seems to be that food eaten late in the day is not digested as effectively and is more likely to lead to weight gain than that eaten earlier. Hence the saying: 'Breakfast like a king, lunch like a prince and dine like a pauper.'

In addition, there is some evidence that men's and women's eating patterns need to be slightly different. Whereas men tend to need three meals a day, women often seem to do better with a larger number of smaller meals. This is not agreed by everyone, but it is important to keep your blood sugar at a reasonable level and this can only be done by ensuring an ongoing supply of energy in your system. This energy is best provided by long-acting complex carbohydrates and, if you do begin to feel hungry between meals, it is probably best to have a small low-fat snack rather than succumb to a food craving as your hunger 'gets the better of you!'

Things to avoid

So far I have talked about things which *are* good for you; what about things which it would be best to avoid?

Caffeine

Found especially in tea, coffee, chocolate and cola drinks, caffeine acts as a stimulant, giving you energy and enthusiasm. Unfortunately, it also acts as a diuretic, making you lose water and leading to dehydration. So avoiding excess caffeine will keep moisture in your body and this will have many benefits, including good skin and higher long-term energy levels. In addition, caffeine can rob your body of essential vitamins and minerals and increase the risk of many health problems. (It has recently been said that tea – both brown and green – can be beneficial as it contains a high level of useful anti-oxidants, but you will have to make up your own mind whether this outweighs the obvious disadvantages of its high caffeine content.)

Highly processed or refined foods

Processed foods may contain high levels of harmful elements and, where possible, it is much better to eat fresh, unprocessed (and, where possible, uncooked) wholefoods.

Colourings and additives

Many people are sensitive to colourings and additives, finding that they can give them headaches, rashes and other side-effects. In children, especially, some additives and colourings can lead to hyperactivity and antisocial behaviour. It is claimed that some additives are essential, for example preservatives in processed foods, but most do not add nutritional value and are best avoided.

There are many publications available on food additives and it is worth reading one of them and then making up your own mind on what to consume.

High-fat products

Fried foods, sausages, crisps, peanuts, unskinned chicken and other products are very high in fat. By reducing your intake of such foods you will take in fewer calories and feel the higher levels of energy that a low-fat diet brings.

Sugar

Sugar has no nutritional value, although it does give a rapid energy boost. Unfortunately, because the energy boost is so rapid, it can stimulate the body to produce higher levels of insulin to help remove the excess sugar from the bloodstream; once the insulin has taken effect, blood sugar drops, often leading to a craving for more sugar, and so a vicious cycle is built up. Avoiding foods with a high added sugar content will help. You might think of using artificial sweeteners instead, but do remember that these are made of chemical compounds which *may* produce unwanted effects in your body. So, because sugar can be obtained naturally from many foods, such as fruits, this is generally a much better option for general health and weight control.

Excess salt

Since so many foods, such as bread, cheese, biscuits and ham, already have added salt, you are unlikely to need much, if any, additional salt in your diet. Of course some salt is necessary but, with the large amount of processed foods we eat, most people get enough without adding more. Added salt is partially an acquired taste and, just as with sugar in tea or coffee, it can be cut out to good effect. Excess salt is implicated in high blood pressure as well as other medical conditions, and it can also lead to water retention, so excessive salt intake is generally to be avoided.

Alcohol

Alcohol depletes the body of some vitamins and minerals by altering their absorption and use, although there is some evidence that a small level of certain kinds of alcohol (wines in particular) can help to reduce certain cholesterol levels. In addition, alcohol tends to be high in calories and it can increase your appetite by lowering your blood sugar levels. Overconsumption of alcohol is not recommended.

Rapid dietary changes

Whatever programme you choose to follow, it is important that you make changes to your diet gradually. Giving your body time to become accustomed to new food regimes makes it easier to adapt.

Eliminating all fat from your diet

It is important to have a balanced diet, with all nutritional elements included. Years ago, diets encouraged people to cut down drastically on carbohydrates; nowadays it is fat which is regarded as the enemy. But the fact is that both carbohydrates and fats are necessary ingredients, although current thinking is that carbohydrates should form the major part of a good diet, with fats being included only at low levels. So maintain a balance in what you eat and cut *down* on fat; do not cut it *out* entirely.

Eliminating things you like from your diet

There is no need to reject any particular food completely. As long as you eat a balanced diet, with plenty of complex carbohydrates to give you sustained energy, you will find that you can still include small amounts of foods which you might have thought of as 'naughty'. And the interesting thing is that, the better your overall eating plan is, the less you will be tempted by foods which are less beneficial.

Food combining

Before we leave this section, you might like to know about some theories about the ways in which foods can be used by your body. Some approaches to eating suggest that certain foods should not be eaten together; this is largely based on the theory that the body digests different foods at different rates and using different enzymes, so that there may be unpleasant consequences of combining foods incorrectly. For example, it is claimed that eating fruit after meat will mean that the fruit breaks down more quickly and, being blocked by the meat eaten previously, is trapped in the stomach, producing gases and causing digestion problems.

Medical opinion seems to be that all food eaten actually ends up in the stomach together and these theories regarding food combining are frequently criticized (apart from the points I have already made about certain vitamins and minerals benefiting from the presence of particular food elements if the body is to utilize them effectively). If you are thinking of embarking on any food regime which involves major changes to your eating habits in such a way, it would be best to do some research yourself before following a programme involving restricted eating.

This part of the chapter has given you guidance about healthy eating. The main guidelines to follow are to eat when you feel hungry, stop when you feel full, eat a balanced diet with plenty of complex carbohydrates to keep you feeling satisfied and plenty of fruit and vegetables to help build defences against illness, allow yourself some of the things you like so that you do not crave them and binge, reduce fat intake to the minimum needed and allow your body time to become re-educated to a healthier pattern of eating.

Exercise

Exercise is a vital part of healthy living and an important element in weight control. Some of the benefits which exercise can bring include better heart and lung functioning, increased flexibility, greater strength, stronger bones and ligaments, lower blood pressure, better muscle condition, improved co-ordination and better handling of stress. Again, only you will know which exercise programme seems best for you, but you might like to consider the following points.

Knowing what kind of exercise to choose

Exercise is anything other than complete immobility. It does not have to be athletics, gymnastics or aerobics; it can also include walking, going up stairs, cleaning the house and dancing. Choosing activities which suit you is likely to keep you motivated and enthusiastic about your programme.

Different kinds of exercise can produce different effects on the body. There are three main ways of exercising – for suppleness, strength and stamina – and the chart overleaf shows how these benefits can be obtained from various exercises.

During exercise, glucose from the food you eat is broken down to provide the energy for your muscles to work, and there are two ways in which your body can work: aerobically and anaerobically.

With aerobic exercise you are generally working a wide range of muscles over an extended period of time, usually at low to moderate levels of activity. Your heart pumps blood round faster, and more oxygen is supplied to your muscles, which benefits your body as a whole and increases your heart's effectiveness. Aerobic exercise involves raising your pulse rate to an optimum level; until you reach that level, although the exercise is still aerobic, it may not be of sufficient intensity to achieve training results and, if you raise your pulse too much, the exercise stops being aerobic as the oxygen supply cannot keep up with your body's needs. You will probably have heard of aerobics classes, which involve

THE HEALTH BENEFITS OF DIFFERENT EXERCERCISE

ACTIVITY	STAMINA	SUPPLENESS	STRENGTH
Aerobics	* * *	* * *	* *
Athletics	* * *	* * *	* *
Badminton	* *	* * *	* *
Circuit training	* * *	* * *	* * *
Cricket	*	* *	*
Cycling	* * * *	* *	* * *
Football	* * *	* * *	* * *
Golf	*	* *	*
Jogging	* * * *	* *	* *
Karate/Judo	*	* *	*
Rowing	* * *	*	* *
Skiing (down hill)	* *	* *	* *
Skipping	* * *	* *	* *
Squash	* * *	* * *	* *
Swimming (hard)	* * * *	* * * *	* * * *
Tennis	* *	* * *	* *
Walking (brisk/hill)	* * *	*	* *
Walking (ramble)	* *	*	*
Weight training	*	* *	* * * *
Yoga	*	* * *	*

* Slight effort   ** Beneficial effort   *** Very good effort   **** Excellent effort

continuous exercises, often to music, to raise your pulse rate and get your body as a whole working well, and other kinds of aerobic activity include running, dancing and rowing.

With anaerobic exercise, you are generally working a limited range of muscles intensively for a short period of time. This kind of exercise is at a higher intensity and raises the heart rate so much that insufficient oxygen is available for your body to work effectively in an aerobic manner. Anaerobic exercise includes weight-lifting, sprinting and jumping.

Both kinds of exercise are good, although they achieve different results; aerobic enhances endurance and anaerobic enhances strength and power. If you wish to lose weight, aerobic exercise is more beneficial, as it may burn more calories from fat and thus reduce the amount of food stored in your body as fat. You must be careful, however, that you do not overdo the level of exercise you take as, once you go into overload, it becomes anaerobic and may be less effective in weight reduction. Aerobic exercise also helps to lower blood pressure, increase HLD ('good cholesterol') levels and improve glucose metabolism, which is a factor in adult-onset diabetes, so it is of great benefit to health generally.

Having said that, however, there are also useful benefits of anaerobic activity. First, exercise such as weight training can increase your muscle quantity and tone; this can improve your posture and help you look slimmer. A further benefit is that, if you do a good deal of anaerobic exercise, you are likely to build more muscle tissue (LBM: Lean Body Mass), and, unlike fat tissue, this increases your metabolic rate (the rate at which you convert food into energy). The American Journal of Clinical Nutrition has stated that an additional 3lb/1.5kg of muscle tissue increases your metabolic rate by 7 per cent. Remember, though, that if you stop exercising, you may lose muscle tissue again, resulting in a slowing again of the rate at which you turn food into energy.

I have said that it helps to raise your pulse rate to an optimum level during exercise. There is a formula used to calculate this level. To find your optimum exercise level you should deduct your age in years from 220. So, if you are 35 years old, you should deduct 35 from 220, which gives you 185. This is your *maximum* heart/pulse rate (MHR). Your optimum exercise rate will vary according to your age and level of fitness. Somewhere between 70 and 80 per cent of MHR is recommended for *reasonably fit* people and the chart opposite gives you an idea of your optimum aerobic exercise level should be.

It is generally recommended that three sessions a week, of at least 20 minutes' duration, where you raise your pulse rate to the extent that you get slightly out of breath but avoid discomfort, are sufficient to produce the increased body function you need to dispose of excess food and keep in good shape. You can, of course, increase this as you become fitter; for most people a maximum amount would be five sessions a week of no more than 45 minutes.

It is also important to consider your 'recovery rate'; the speed with which your pulse rate comes back to its 'resting' level after exercise is another indicator of your general fitness level.

You can buy small devices which will measure your pulse rate and tell you the level at which you are

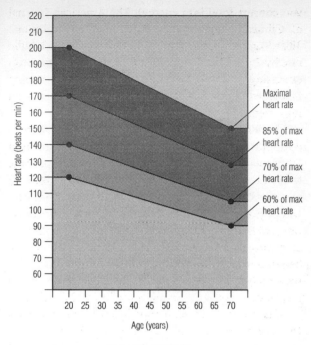

Maximal Heart Rate Guide

exercising, or you can simply take your pulse yourself from time to time. The advantage of the pulse monitors is that you do not have to keep stopping if you want to check your pulse rate.

To take your own pulse, place the tips of your three middle fingers on the opposite wrist and press until you feel a pulse. The place to feel is on the inside of the wrist, approximately in line with your first finger and below the base of your thumb. Once you can feel the pulse, look at a watch and count how many beats there are in a ten-second period; then multiply by six and this will give you your pulse rate (beats per minute).

Aim to increase your pulse rate when exercising in line with the recommended level for your age and remember that the fitter you are the more your resting pulse rate (the rate at which your pulse goes when you are inactive) is likely to drop.

Understanding the value of different kinds of exercise

Although this book has not focused on calorie counting, it is useful to know how different activities compare in terms of the energy they use up when you do them. The following chart has been compiled from various sources and gives you an idea of how useful some common activities can be in your programme.

The chart shows the approximate number of calories burned in ten minutes of continuous activity. Of course,

Activity	Calories burned in 10 minutes
Aerobic dancing	74
Badminton	70
Cycling	65
Dancing	50
Gardening	50
Mowing the lawn	60
Riding	58
Running	110
Squash	106
Swimming	110
Table tennis	43
Tennis	65
Vacuuming	40
Walking downhill	55
Walking uphill/stairs	160

you can do the activities at different levels of effort, so the figures below are for average levels of exertion. Most of the figures are given for a person weighing around 140lb/64 kg; the more you weigh, the more calories you will burn with any given activity (apart from swimming, which uses the same regardless of your weight out of the water), so the chart is simply a guide to energy consumption. And also remember that each person will have his or her own way of doing exercises so, again, the amounts of energy used will vary.

All activities do not produce the same health and fitness benefits. For example, while swimming is excellent for general fitness, weight-bearing exercise such as walking is much more effective for maintaining bone density. So select your activities according to what you enjoy, what you can fit into your lifestyle and what results you want them to achieve.

You do not need to do any specialized kinds of exercise to get fit. Some of the most useful things you can do can be done in and around your home. For example, vacuuming the house will exercise a range of muscles and, if you do it rapidly, will be aerobic exercise. Going up and down stairs will have a similar effect. You can do abdominal (stomach) firming exercises easily through sit-ups (but make sure you do them correctly in order to avoid strain on your back). Dancing to music at home is also excellent exercise. If you want to do muscle-strengthening exercises you can use household objects, for example bags of sugar or small cans of food, as weights (but do get advice first on using weights correctly). You can also get a skipping rope to use in the garden or, if you want to go further, invest in a mini-trampoline, exercise bike or small multi-gym which you can use at home. Some of this equipment folds away to store, but do be careful to get equipment which functions well, is comfortable to use and is well balanced and stable. There are many sources of advice on home equipment, including fitness magazines, personal trainers and sports organizations.

Setting realistic goals

Whatever exercise you choose, it is important to set yourself goals which are realistic and which you will pursue enthusiastically. I discussed goal setting in chapter 4, so all I need say here is that having a goal will help keep you on track and help you check how well you are doing.

It is important to remember that we all have our own individual body proportions, including our height, the relative width of our shoulders and hips, the length of our necks, arms and legs, the size of our hands and feet, the shape of our faces and so forth. It is important to understand that these proportions cannot, in the normal course of events, be changed and that to aspire to the body shape of another person is a fruitless endeavour. Accepting your own unique shape is as important as acknowledging your own unique personality.

Listening to your body

This is an essential element in successful exercising. How many times have you seen people overdoing things because they have not taken notice of what their body was telling them. If you pay attention, you will be able to develop the ability to notice when the time is right for you to exercise and when it is right to slow down or to stop.

If you take notice of it, your body will tell you what to do by giving you signals, which can include:

- tiredness
- aching muscles
- cramp
- stiffness
- loss of concentration
- overheating
- becoming chilled
- getting breathless

By noticing these signals you can adjust what you do to keep at a suitable pace for your own ability and energy levels. The more you pay attention in this way, the better you will become at determining whether to continue or to stop.

Of course there will be times when, although you think you feel tired, some activity will actually help you re-energize yourself, but you should be careful to assess carefully whether this is the case or whether you are actually too tired to exercise. Similarly, if you are exercising and begin to feel stiff or uncomfortable, it is probably best to stop for the time being and rest. Do not, on any account, give in to pressure by friends or instructors to continue if you are convinced that you have had enough. A few moments too much can mean a good deal of time off recuperating. And if at any time you get pains in your chest when exercising stop immediately and, if they persist after you have stopped the exercise, go to see your doctor.

Varying what you do

Although exercise is important, many people find that they can get bored with repeating the same kind of activities for long periods. Building flexibility into your exercise programme is important, both to avoid boredom and to make the most of the activities you pursue. Because muscle fibres need a period of rest in order to become strong, it helps to rotate your programme so as to do activities which exercise different parts of your body at different times. This is more important if you do a large amount of exercise; with mild exercise it is less important as you will be putting less strain on any particular muscle group at any particular time but, if you are keen to build up your efforts, then a varied schedule will probably work best for you.

Exercising at the right level

Each person has an optimum range of activity and the chart on page 183 suggests exercise pulse rates for different ages. If you have any particular health problems which could mean that raising your pulse rate should be avoided, do check with your doctor before starting and, if you have not taken regular exercise for some time, it is probably wisest to have a medical check-up before you do anything strenuous. It is also important to get medical advice before starting exercise if you have heart problems, chest pains, high blood pressure, asthma, bronchitis, back trouble, arthritis or diabetes, or are just recovering from an illness or operation.

Once you do start to exercise, you may find that using a pulse rate monitor helps you check that you are exercising within an appropriate range, although your body will more often than not give you much the same information without the expense of an additional piece of equipment. However, monitors can help, especially at the early stages of a programme to let you know how you are doing or, if you are very advanced, to make sure you are adequately challenged by your exercise programme or are keeping within the goal levels you have set yourself.

Warming up

Whatever exercise you do, it is important to take some time at the start and end of a session to warm up and to cool down. There are two things you can do which will help. First, right at the start of each session take a few minutes to do gentle warm-up exercises such as five minutes on an exercise bike, or steady walking, which will increase your temperature and help loosen your joints. After you have done this, you can then do stretching exercises, which may help prevent strain or injury during your workout. You should reduce your activity gradually and do stretching exercises again at the end of your session, which will help avoid stiffness after exercising. You should make sure you stretch all the major muscle groups in your body during stretching sessions. For advice on suitable warm-up and stretching exercises you should consult a fitness expert; *see* Useful Addresses at the end of this book.

Building in progressive effort

Your body can easily get used to any particular level of effort. You may take up an exercise which feels hard at the time but, after a week or so, it may feel really easy. When it becomes easy it is less of a challenge to your body, so regularly upgrading the level of effort you put in is important. If you are working with a personal trainer, or attending supervised sessions, you will be able to get professional advice on how to do this.

Maintaining your programme of exercise

Exercise helps you build strong and flexible muscles, but muscle tissue is easily lost. If you have a period of inactivity, even of a few days, you quickly lose the strength and tone you have built up previously. So to keep in good shape it is important to maintain a regular programme of activity. This is why it is so important to choose activities which you enjoy; it makes it so much easier for you to keep to your programme and to maintain your interest.

Classes and personal trainers

More and more people are turning to organized sessions to help them exercise. Leisure centres and gyms are springing up and offering a wider range of services to their customers. Some of the things you may come across in such places are aerobics classes (designed to raise your pulse rate and strengthen your heart), circuit training (mainly designed to develop strength, body tone and power), product-based training (such as step or slide programmes)and aqua-aerobics (aerobic exercises carried out in a swimming pool).

An alternative to organized classes is to get together with a friend and help each other as you progress, or to make use of the services of a personal trainer. A personal trainer is someone with specialist training and experience of fitness and exercise, who can help you by designing, and supporting you in, a personal programme of exercise activity (sometimes advice is given on diet too).

For many people a personal trainer is a good investment, both from the point of view of professional advice and from the point of view of motivation and morale boosting when needed. And do remember, personal trainers will be able to come to your home if you wish, so you do not have to work out in front of other people in a leisure centre or gym. To find a personal trainer, or exercise class, see Useful Addresses at the end of this book.

Some things to avoid

As with food, there are certain elements of exercise which are best avoided.

Exercising immediately after eating

You need some food in your body to supply energy for exercise, but you should avoid strenuous exercise immediately after eating because exercise can divert needed blood away from your digestive system, where it is required after a meal. Gentle walking after a meal is a good activity, and beneficial, but wait at least two hours before doing anything more strenuous, particularly swimming as you could get cramps if you swim soon after eating.

Exercising when you are not up to it

If you listen to your body, as I mentioned above, you will know when not to do exercise. By pacing yourself you will make the most of the time you do spend on exercising.

Using unfamiliar equipment

You may want to go to a gym or leisure centre to exercise. If you do, make sure you have a proper induction session showing you exactly how to use the various items of equipment. It is possible to cause strain or injury if you use equipment incorrectly or at too high a level of effort. Always get professional advice before starting. You might also check that the centre has insurance cover, in the unlikely event that you sustain an injury while using their equipment.

Doing harmful exercises

Even in this health-conscious age, there are still books, tapes and professional trainers that recommend undertaking exercises which are likely to be harmful. Usually such exercises put undue strain on the back or neck, or involve using muscles within very limited ranges of movement, which can lead to shortening and tightening of the muscle fibres. If you feel at all uncomfortable during any form of exercise, stop doing it and discuss it with someone who is well informed. It may be that the exercise itself is not a good one, or it may simply be that your technique is not correct and you need help.

Therapies

There are many processes, often referred to as complementary therapies, which can help you in keeping your body in good condition. I will describe some of these here. If you would like to find a person who specializes in one of these areas, refer to Useful Addresses at the end of the book.

Massage

Massage stimulates the body to function well. In particular, it stimulates the lymphatic system, which is responsible for eliminating waste products from the body; it also helps with relaxation, and research indicates that it enhances the functioning of the immune system. There are many forms of massage, including aromatherapy, a very mild form which uses scented oils to soothe, energize or help break down fatty tissue and impurities. It is interesting to note that many forward-thinking employers now allow trained people to come to their premises and offer neck and shoulder massage to staff at their place of work; if you are fortunate enough to work in such a place, do make the most of the facilities offered.

Detoxification

It is generally believed that the body accumulates toxins, including by-products of its functioning such as lactic acid and adrenalin, and also by-products of such things as overprocessed foods, air pollution etc. If these toxins are not excreted normally, they can build up within the body. Detoxification leads to better health and a better functioning metabolism. Although some people disagree that it is necessary to detoxify, it can do no harm to follow the guidelines.

Detoxification includes a range of activities, the most common of which are: eating a low-fat, high-fibre diet with plenty of fresh foods, including fruit, vegetables and wholegrains; drinking a reasonable quantity of fresh water; having massages, saunas or Turkish baths; and occasional mild fasting.

It is claimed that detoxification (particularly if short periods of fasting are involved) may cause symptoms such as headaches and facial spots in the very short term, but that this is a sign that the body is eliminating harmful wastes. If you are interested in this topic, there are many books available on it.

Health resorts

These are places where you can take advantage of various services and activities. They offer such facilities as swimming pools, spas, hydros, beauty salons, massage, flotation tanks for relaxation, expert advice on nutrition, diet and exercise, health checks, low-calorie meals, sports and gymnastic facilities, exercise classes, and talks on relevant subjects. They are excellent for relaxation and giving your programme a boost, and you may find that a few days at one is a good investment (and it *is* likely to be an investment; health resorts do not generally offer a low-cost service).

The Alexander technique and Feldenkrais

These two approaches are very helpful in a weight-control programme as they re-educate you in how to sit, stand and move in a balanced way. As you lose weight, you will find it useful to have guidance on good body use so that you can make the most of your new shape and size. The Alexander technique is a system of body alignment and balance, usually carried out in one-to-one sessions with a teacher, which shows you how to use your body well and avoid bad habits in posture and movement. Alexander lessons usually last around three-quarters of an hour, and a course of treatments, with continuing follow-up sessions, is generally recommended. A similar approach to Alexander is Feldenkrais, which also involves learning to use the body by developing awareness through movement.

194

Stress-management techniques

The avoidance or removal of stress is vital to healthy living. Although many of us lead pressured lives and thrive on them, stress is different and its presence encourages the body to develop both physical and mental ailments. Remaining free of stress will help you in managing and keeping to your programme.

There are many techniques available for alleviating stress, including relaxation, meditation, hypnosis (and self-hypnosis), hobbies and sports. It has been reported that an aid to avoiding stress is to take regular breaks. *The Twenty Minute Break* by Ernest Rossi, is excellent on this.

Sleep, rest and relaxation

This is not really a therapy but it is certainly therapeutic. Getting enough sleep and rest will help you with your programme, as it is important to have enough energy to be able to function effectively and do those things you need to in order to lose weight. It is helpful to have regular breaks during the day, to relax both mentally and physically. If possible, a 20-minute break every hour and a half is ideal, but shorter breaks will do if you cannot manage more. By listening to your body you will begin to recognize when it needs a break (typical signs are tiredness, lack of concentration, hunger, yawning and needing to go to the lavatory). When you notice these signs it is time for a break. Take a little time to move around, change the focus of your eyes (if you have been doing close work then look at some things in the distance to give your eyes a rest), close your eyes if possible and, if you can, lie down and empty your mind for a while. You will find this really beneficial and a good aid to both relaxation and overall performance.

This chapter has given you information about a whole range of lifestyle activities. Do explore any aspects of it which you think will be personally useful; the attention you give to both your body and your mind will help you create and maintain a healthy and positive lifestyle.

Conclusion

Now that you have reached the end of the book you will have found out how to achieve your own personal weight-control programme. The techniques I have been describing have been shown to be effective with many people in all walks of life. The important thing is for you to have a real commitment to losing weight and to take the time to understand what works best for you.

Whatever your past views on your ability to lose weight, let me remind you once again: everyone can lose weight if they do the right things. Whatever your present size, age, temperament and lifestyle, there will be an approach which works for you – you just need to persevere. If you do have the odd setback, remember that it just shows you are human. You do have the ability to see past it, keep your future goals in mind and continue on the right track.

Because everyone is different, the way you put the ideas from this book into practice will be very personal to you. You may have friends who are also concerned about their weight; remember that they are different and, although your approach works for you, something different may be needed for them. But whatever your personal approach, it will be aided enormously by harnessing the power of your mind to get you to where you want to be.

You may also find that there are other areas of your life which you wish to change, and the processes you have read about here will help with these too. You can use the same processes of goal setting, thinking positively and taking action to get results. The important thing to remember is that you are the only one who can make it real. You can read, talk to other people, get information and plan what to do; but in the end it is your own efforts which will bring you the results you desire.

So really make up your mind to do well and see just how successful you can be. And when you have achieved your goals, if you feel like writing to let me know, I would be delighted to hear from you; I enjoy collecting success stories.

APPENDIX:
Facts About Weight

This appendix gives you some background information to the processes covered in this book. Although it is not essential to read, I think you will find many of the facts presented here fascinating and useful.

How big is the problem?

Many people are concerned about their weight. Weight gains seem to be on the increase. In the past 10–15 years, there has been a rapid increase in weight gains all round the world, especially in countries where incomes are high and food supplies are plentiful and varied.

In the UK and the USA, around half the total population is overweight (in the UK almost half the adult women take a dress size of 16 or over), and studies have shown that one in four Americans and around one in five British people are clinically obese (*see* page 200 for a definition of obesity). In the UK, the average woman is 9lb/4kg heavier now than in 1980 (*Top Santé* magazine, July 1998). And weight gains do not just apply to people either; a recent TV programme in the UK showed that a third of the nation's pet dogs were obese too!

A worrying fact about weight is that there is an increasing trend towards children and young people becoming overweight. Recent research showed that one in 20 children in the UK is seriously overweight and 20 per cent of children in the UK face health risks as adults because of their weight level. The increasing use of cars to take children to and from school and other activities and the decrease in organized sports activities in schools, both contribute to the problem. There is also evidence that if fat is accumulated early in life it is more likely to persist later on and can be difficult to shift; so helping children to stay fit and healthy is a long-term investment in their future.

Defining obesity

There is a difference between just being overweight and being obese, or severely overweight. Being overweight is simply weighing more than is average for your height, whereas obesity is defined rather differently. Obesity is extreme overweight, and is considered by doctors to be a chronic condition and a leading cause of heart disease, diabetes and cancer. In addition, women who diet excessively and take little exercise run increased risks of osteoporosis (or thinning of the bones). Although you *can* be overweight and still fit, it is said that an obese person has a 30 per cent higher risk of dying in any given year (*Top Santé* magazine, July 1998). Interestingly, in those countries where research has been carried out, the results show that men are more likely to be overweight, whereas women are more likely to be obese.

It is hard to get agreement on how to define obesity, as different countries have their own definitions. However there is one measure which has gained considerable agreement, the Body Mass Index (BMI).

The BMI is an index of weight in relation to height and is calculated by taking your weight (in kilograms) and dividing it by the square of your height (in metres). This gives you a figure which then shows whether you are overweight. This formula can be used by everyone, men and women, although it should not be applied to children, pregnant women or people with very high muscle development, such as athletes.

The varying ranges of weight are shown below:

Category	BMI
Underweight	under 20
Normal weight	20–24.9
Overweight	25–29.9
Obese	30–39.9
Severely obese	40 and over

Average weights for the healthy person

It is possible to assess whether your weight falls within 'normal' ranges by looking at charts, and one such chart is shown overleaf. You should remember a number of facts, though, when using weight charts. The first is that weight can vary according to bone density (how heavy your bones are) and according to your sex (men generally weigh more than women at any particular height). Secondly, weight charts do not take into account the relative amount of fat you are carrying so, as I have explained below, you can weigh a 'correct' amount, but still carry a lot of fat rather than muscle tissue. And thirdly, the people on whom these charts were originally based were not a typical cross-section of the population; they were simply people chosen by a life insurance company as being long-lived. They only reported their weights once and were not actually measured, and no account was taken of any health problems or weight gains occurring after the initial weight was reported.

Bearing all this in mind, here is a sample table but please use it only as a *general* guide, not an absolute one.

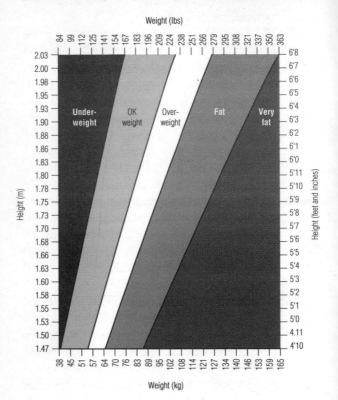

Knowing how much excess weight you are carrying

Your body has both fat and lean muscle tissue and they weigh different amounts. Fat weighs less than lean muscle. Because of this, you can be very heavy yet have little fat, or be within the 'normal' weight range for your height, yet carry a lot of fat on your body. For example, many people who are extremely fit, such as professional athletes, are actually quite heavy for their height, yet carry little or no excess fat.

This also means that it is not enough simply to know your overall weight, as one person may be heavier than another yet less fat, because of carrying more lean tissue. And do remember, too, that when you exercise more, although you will lose fat, your muscle tissue will weigh more, so overall weight loss is a fairly complex process.

There is also a difference in the amount of fat carried by men and women, with women generally having higher proportions of body fat. (A healthy range for men is 12–17 per cent fat and for women 18–22 per cent fat) (American College of Sports Medicine). So, although the chart opposite is basically correct, you still need to take into account your sex and your general level of fitness and body tone when considering how overweight you are.

Finally, water retention can contribute to overall weight. Women may have increased levels of water in their bodies at certain times of the month. Moreover, because you need a certain amount of water for general hydration, if you drink too little your body thinks it is being deprived of fluid and tends to hang on to the water it has. So by drinking adequate amounts of water each day, surprisingly you are likely to have less water retention rather than more. And remember that if you do have water retention, the first stage of a weight-loss programme may result in water loss before your body fat begins to be reduced.

Understanding the importance of where your fat is located

Where you store fat in your body is important. In particular, fat accumulation around your stomach is more of a problem than other areas, because fat around your waist can get into the bloodstream more easily, leading to an increased risk of heart disease and diabetes in some people.

Men are more likely to store fat around their stomachs, but it does also happen in women, especially if they are very overweight. Sometimes people refer to body shapes as 'apple' and 'pear', with 'apples' having much of their fat around their stomachs (rounded like an apple; more common in men) and 'pears' having much of their fat around their hips and thighs (pear shaped, with narrow shoulders; more common in women). Again, there is a formula for calculating whether you are an 'apple' or a 'pear' and, if you are becoming apple shaped, it is definitely time to make a change in your lifestyle if you wish to remain fit and healthy.

To calculate whether you are apple shaped, you will need to use what is known as the WHR (waist-to-hip ratio). To do this, you need to divide your waist measurement by your hip measurement. Measure your waist at the smallest point between your ribcage and your belly button; measure your hip at the largest point in your hip/buttock area. Different sources quote slightly different figures as indicating apple shapes, but in general if you are a woman and the figure is over 0.85 you are apple shaped and if you are a man and the figure is above 0.95 you are apple shaped.

The good news is that, if you are apple shaped, it is

easier for you to lose weight than if you are pear shaped, as fat stored around your abdomen tends to be easier to lose than fat around your hips, buttocks and thighs. As the health risks of excess fat around your stomach are quite significant, do make a real effort to reduce if this figure is high for you.

Measures of food intake

Finally, you might like to know about some different ways of estimating the impact of what you are eating. There are three main ways in which you can assess your food intake; theses are:

Counting calories

A calorie is a unit of energy. All food gives you energy and the amount of energy it gives you is counted in calories. Calorie counting is the traditional way of assessing your food intake and, in the past, most diet plans advised you to measure the calorie content of your food and then limit your total calorie intake to certain levels if you wished to lose weight. There are disadvantages to this approach because, while you will know how many calories you are taking in, you don't know what kind of calories they are. For example, you could consume 500 calories in pure sugar, which would not provide you with any nutrients, or you could consume 500 calories in fresh vegetables, which would give you both energy and nutritional value. So calorie counting alone does not ensure a balanced diet – it is also very time consuming and makes you think about food all the time.

Counting fats

Another way of assessing your food is by using 'fat units'. Many foods contain fats and there are ways of assessing the relative fat content of different foods. As low-fat diets are now generally recommended, choosing your food in terms of its fat level is sensible; remembering that, for the same weight of food, fat has over twice the calories of protein or carbohydrate. As an example, a cup of full-fat milk has ten fat units, semi-skimmed has four, skimmed has none and soya milk has five; 4oz (112gms) chicken with skin has nineteen, whereas without skin it has four; and 4oz (112gms) of cabbage, carrot or boiled or baked potato has none (Figures taken from *The Complete Fat Counter* by Peter Cox and Peggy Brusseau, Bloomsday, 1998.) It is important to have some fat in your diet but, by limiting your intake of food with a high fat unit count, you can really help your programme along.

Counting sugars

And another way of assessing your food is by considering its sugar content. Many foods contain sugar and the sugar levels in food can be assessed by noting what is called the 'Glycaemic Index' – GI for short. Each food has a figure on the Glycaemic Index (from 0 to 100), depending on the extent to which the food will raise blood sugar levels. High index foods give you an initial boost, but then stimulate insulin production to remove the excess sugar from your system. This tends to make your blood sugar drop and make you feel hungry. Low index foods give you a more sustained energy boost and are very helpful in a weight control programme as they keep you feeling satisfied for longer. So the high index foods break down the quickest during digestion, while the low index foods are more slowly digested.

While simple carbohydrates are more likely to have a high GI figure some complex carbohydrates also do. Although complex carbohydrates are generally good in a weight-control programme, certain ones are more likely to keep your hunger at bay for longer and some simple carbohydrates can also have a similar effect. As an example, pasta, porridge and lentils are digested slowly, while many breakfast cereals are quickly absorbed into your system. The GI figure for some of these foods are as follows: lentils 29, yoghurt 33, porridge 42, white bread 70, wholemeal breakfast cereal 77, baked potato 85. (Figures taken from *The GI Factor: the Glycaemic Index Solution* by Tony Leeds and J B Miller, Hodder, 1998.)

So, not all foods are equal in terms of their value in your diet. A balanced diet, with plenty of all the major food elements and groups, is the best for healthy living. In addition, if you keep your diet low in foods with substantial fat and sugar elements, you will be helping your body make the most of its nutrition and helping yourself lead a healthy, fit and enjoyable life.

Bibliography

Andreas, Connirae and Steve, *Heart of the Mind*, Real People Press, 1989

Batmanghelidj, F, *Your Body's Many Cries For Water*, The Therapist Ltd, 1994

Charvet, Shelle Rose, *Words That Change Minds*, Kendall/Hunt Publishing, 1997

Harris, Carol, *The Elements of NLP*, Element Books, Shaftesbury, 1998

Maltz, Maxwell, *Psycho-Cybernetics*, Prentice-Hall, Englewood Cliffs, USA, 1960

Robbins, Anthony, *Unlimited Power*, Simon & Schuster, London, 1988

Rossi, Ernest Lawrence, *The Twenty Minute Break*, Palisades Gateway, 1991

AUDIOTAPES

Harris, Carol, *Success in Mind* series, 1995: *Super Slimming, Super Self, Creating a Good Impression, Handling Social Situations, Active Job Seeking*. Available direct from Management Magic, PO Box 47, Welshpool, Powys, SY21 7NX.

Credits

Some of the motivational patterns in this book have been based on what are known in NLP as meta-programmes developed by David Gordon and Leslie Cameron-Bondler. Rodger Bailey and Shelle Rose Charvet have published material on this (the LAB profile and the book *Words That Change Minds* – *see* opposite). Thanks are also given to Setform Ltd, Chartex Products International Ltd, and the Health Education Authority for permission to use their charts.

Useful Addresses

AUSTRALIA

Australian Feldenkrais Guild
PO Box 285
Ashfield
NSW 2132
Tel: 8 8269 7783

**Australian Fitness Accreditation Council
(AFAC)**
PO Box 2392V
Melbourne
Tel: 3 9655 5387

Australian Health Care Association
PO Box 54
Deakin West
ACT 2600
Tel: 6285 1488

Australian Institute of Yoga Therapy
7/71 Ormond Road
Elwood
Victoria 3184
Tel: 9525 6951

Australian Nutrition Foundation
1/3 Derwent Street
Glebe
NSW 2037
Tel: 9442 3081

Australian Society of Teachers of the Alexander Technique (AUSTAT)
PO Box 716
Darlinghurst
NSW 2010
Tel: 008 339 571

National Therapists Association
PO Box 856
Caloundra
Queensland 4551
Tel: 5491 9850

CANADA

Canadian Association of Fitness Professionals (CAN FIT PRO)
Galleria London
355 Wellington Street
PO Box 122, London
Ontario N6A 3N7
Tel: 905 305 8450

Canadian Society of Teachers of the Alexander Technique (CANSTAT)
1472 East St Joseph Boulevard
Apt No 4, Montreal
Quebec H2J IM5
Tel: 514 522 9230

NEW ZEALAND

New Zealand Feldenkrais Guild
PO Box 46296
Herne Bay
Auckland
Tel: 64 9 378 8091

SOUTH AFRICA

South African Aerobics Federation
Daniella Clack
PO Box 30
Gallo Manor 2052
Tel: 11 802 2378

South African Society of Teachers of the Alexander Technique (SASTAT)
17 Ash Street
Observatory 7925
Cape Town
Tel: 021 47 0436

UK

Aerobics and Fitness Organisation of Great Britain
Garrick House
9 High Street
Glinton
Peterborough
Cambs PE6 7JP
Tel: 01733 252543

Association of Reflexologists
27 Old Gloucester Street
London WC1V 3XX
Tel: 08705 673320

Association of Personal Trainers
Suite 2
8 Bedford Court
London WC2E 9LU
Tel: 0171 379 5552

Exercise Association of England
Unit 4
Angel Gate
City Road
London EC1V 2PT
Tel: 0171 278 0811

Feldenkrais Guild UK
PO Box 370
London N10 3XA
Tel: 07000 785 506

Health Education Authority
Treveyan House,
30 Great Peter Street
London SW1P 2HW
Tel: 0171 222 5300

Institute for Complementary Medicine
15 Tavern Quay
London SE16 1AA
Tel: 0171 237 5165

Institute for Optimum Nutrition
Blades Court
Deodar Road
London SW15 2NU
Tel: 0181 877 9993

Kinesiology Federation
PO Box 83
Sheffield S7 2YN
Tel: 0114 281 4064

The Professional Association of Alexander Teachers
Carol Taylor (Secretary – from 4/99)
20 High Street
Norton
Stockton-on-Tees
Cleveland TS20 1DN
Tel: 01642 363542

Society of Teachers of the Alexander Technique
20 London House
266 Fulham Road
London SW10 9EL
Tel: 0171 351 0828

214

USA

Aerobics and Fitness Association of America (AFAA)
15250 Ventura Boulevard
Sherman Oaks
California 91403
Tel: 818 9050040
(International organization with branches in over 70 countries.)

American Council on Exercise
5820 Oberlin Drive
Suite 102
San Diego
CA 92121-3787
Tel: 619 535 8227

American Medical Association (AMA)
515N, State St
Chicago
Il 60610
Tel: 001 312 464 5000

Feldenkrais Guild of North America
PO Box 489
Albany
OR

215

International Dance and Exercise Association (IDEA)
6190 Cornerstone Ct E
Suite 204
San Diego
California 92121-3773
Tel: 619 535 8979

International Life Sciences Institute (ILSI)
1126 Sixteenth Street NW
Suite 300
Washington DC 20036
Tel: 202 659 0074
(And branches worldwide including Australasia, Europe, Japan, and South Africa.)

North American Society of Teachers of the Alexander Technique (NASTAT)
3010 Hennepin Avenue South
Suite 10
Minneapolis
MIN 55408
Tel: 612 824 5066
(free call within USA: 800 473 0620)

INDEX